Procedure Manual for
Pediatric Nursing

Niyati Das

RN RM MSc Nursing
Professor cum Vice Principal
Kalinga Institute of Nursing Sciences
KIIT (deemed to be) University, Bhubaneswar, Odisha

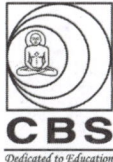

CBS
Dedicated to Education

CBS Publishers and Distributors Pvt Ltd

• New Delhi • Bengaluru • Chennai • Kochi • Kolkata • Mumbai
• Hyderabad • Nagpur • Patna • Pune • Vijayawada

Procedure Manual for

Pediatric Nursing

ISBN: 978-93-88108-86-7

Copyright © Publishers

First Edition: 2018

All rights reserved. No part of this book may be reproduced or transmitted in any form or by any means, electronic or mechanical, including photocopying, recording, or any information storage and retrieval system without permission, in writing, from the publishers.

Published by **Satish Kumar Jain** and produced by **Varun Jain** for

CBS Publishers and Distributors Pvt Ltd

4819/XI Prahlad Street, 24 Ansari Road, Daryaganj, New Delhi 110 002, India.
Ph: 23289259, 23266861, 23266867   Website: www.cbspd.com
Fax: 011-23243014
e-mail: delhi@cbspd.com; cbspubs@airtelmail.in.
Corporate Office: 204 FIE, Industrial Area, Patparganj, Delhi 110 092
Ph: 4934 4934   Fax: 4934 4935
e-mail: bhupesharora@cbspd.com

Branches

- **Bengaluru:** Seema House 2975, 17th Cross, K.R. Road,
  Banasankari 2nd Stage, Bengaluru 560 070, Karnataka
  Ph: +91-80-26771678/79   Fax: +91-80-26771680
  e-mail: bangalore@cbspd.com

- **Chennai:** No. 7, Subbaraya Street, Shenoy Nagar, Chennai 600 030, Tamil Nadu
  Ph: +91-44-42032115   Fax: +91-44-42032115
  e-mail: chennai@cbspd.com

- **Kochi:** Ashana House, 39/1904, AM Thomas Road, Valanjambalam, Eranakulam 682 018, Kochi, Kerala
  Ph: +91-484-4059061-62-64-65   Fax: +91-484-4059065
  e-mail: kochi@cbspd.com

- **Kolkata:** No. 6/B, Ground Floor, Rameswar Shaw Road, Kolkata-700014 (West Bengal), India
  Ph: +91-33-2289-1126, 2289-1127
  e-mail: kolkata@cbspd.com

- **Mumbai:** 83-C, Dr E Moses Road, Worli, Mumbai-400018, Maharashtra
  Ph: +91-22-24902340/41   Fax: +91-22-24902342
  e-mail: mumbai@cbspd.com

Representatives

- Hyderabad   +91-9885175004
- Vijaywada   +91-74069-04007
- Nagpur   +91-9021734563
- Mangalore +91-9741432102
- Patna   +91-9334159340

Printed At : Goyal Offset Printers

From Publisher's Desk

"Gaining knowledge is the first step to wisdom. Sharing it is the first step to humanity."

The above mentioned lines form the foundation stone of CBS publishers and Distributors Pvt Ltd, the flag bearer in medical publishing. Headquartered in New Delhi, the national capital of India, CBS was established in the year 1972 and it has expanded its roots to grow as a pioneer in the field of medical publishing in Asia. CBS is one of the largest and the fastest growing publishers of medical books in Southeast Asia. We are partners in the education of undergraduate and postgraduate students for we believe in nurturing the brains of medicos since the beginning of their careers in medicine. CBS joins the hands with the medical students as their first choice since the very moment they enter the college with BD Chaurasia's Human Anatomy and CC Chatterjee's Human Physiology. CBS is the proud owner of many bestselling titles like OP Ghai's Textbook of Pediatrics, Manipal's Surgery, KD Chatterjee's Textbook of Parasitology, and the list goes on. CBS has successfully partnered in sculpting the careers of millions of medicos across the world.

After successfully establishing an important place in the careers of medical and allied sciences' students for almost four decades, it is our great privilege to announce the launch of "CBS Nursing Knowledge Tree" – a novel endeavor to partner with the Nursing fraternity in Quality Education.

Vision and Mission of CBS Nursing Knowledge Tree

CBS Nursing Knowledge Tree is conceptualized with a vision of being the first of its kind to bring the best quality books for education of Nurses. Keeping in mind the changing trends in the Nursing Education, we at CBS have taken up a mission to bring student-friendly and syllabus-based books written by Subject Experts from PAN India without compromising on the Quality of content and presenting it in a Unique manner.

Foundation Stones of CBS Nursing Knowledge Tree

- **Strong editorial support by the leading subject experts and faculties in Nursing from PAN India.** Every manuscript/proposal that is received is critically reviewed by our Editorial Board at various levels to ensure the Quality of content. A book is published only after all the parameters in our process management are satisfied.
- **Special care taken to publish Plagiarism-free matter.** With the copyright laws being highly strict these days, we at CBS are paying extra attention at various stages of publishing a book to crosscheck and avoid any copyright infringement.
- **Books authored by Subject Experts and Senior Faculties all over India.** Every title owned by CBS Nursing Knowledge Tree is written by the senior-most faculties and subject masters from every nook and corner of the country to provide them a bigger platform to share their knowledge and experience amongst budding nursing fraternity.
- **All the books developed as per INC syllabus and needs of the students without compromising on the Quality of the content.** Often students complain that some books are either not covering the complete syllabus or have too much content as compared to the syllabus. In this series, extra care is being taken to develop books strictly as per INC syllabus in the most student-friendly manner.
- **All books being reviewed by Top-notch faculties and Subject Experts to maintain high standards of Quality.** Every title goes through tough grilling regarding the content and the overall presentation by various top subject experts as reviewers. This ensures that only the Quality content gets published.
- **Best International standard layouts for every book.** Every title in CBS Nursing Knowledge Tree is designed and formatted in the best layouts of international standards because we strongly believe that every book deserves to be treated the Best!
- **Additional and Unique features given with every title.** Every title is accompanied by one or the other additional feature to complement the learning of students like—*Workbook, DVD, Last Minute Revision Notes*. We have also included many features like *How to make Most out of this Book, Assess Yourself* that contains questions and MCQs and other special boxes according to the need of the content.

Let's Join Our Hands Together

We can only bring the change that we want to see in Nursing Education with the support and cooperation of leading faculties in all Nursing specialties. If you envision the same, we are happy to welcome you to our panel of contributors and reviewers and let's take up this mission together of creating a Change in Nursing Education.

We crave cooperation from all the students and faculties to provide their genuine feedback on the quality of the books and how we can improve upon the deficiencies in future on the following email id: cbsvpdesk@yahoo.com. Constructive criticism with concrete suggestions for improvement for all our books will be highly appreciated.

Expanding Horizons

We are also highly active in attending various National Level Conferences and Meets organized by various Nursing Societies. We are keenly working to expand our horizons of associations by participating in conferences organized by **SOCHNI, ISPN, NRSI, ICMR, SOMI,** etc. every year. CBS has always been a forerunner and a big supporter of all National level Nursing Conferences. *If you have any National and State level conference proposals, we are happy to be the part of these conferences.*

Being Social is Our Aspiration

In this era of Social Media, we are happy being social as well by bringing you our Facebook page **facebook.com/ cbsnursingtree** of "CBS Nursing Knowledge Tree" to expand our reach to the maximum people in Nursing. It is a platform purely dedicated to bring the important aspects and latest updates and developments in various domains and fields of Nursing. It will be our privilege if you could connect with us and share your knowledge and experiences as well on our Facebook page.

I would like to invite all the readers to come and join us on our facebook page and share some input, information and literature.

With this vision and above features we are happy to announce the release of **Procedure Manual for Pediatric Nursing** by **Ms Niyati Das.**

This **Procedure Manual** has been written keeping in mind the need and wants of GNM, Post Basic Bsc, Basic BSc and MSc nursing students.

I look forward that you enjoy the reading of this book!

Bhupesh Arora

Vice President-Publishing and Marketing
(NURSING Division)
CBS Publishers and Distributors (Delhi) Pvt. Ltd.
Email: bhupesharora@cbspd.com
Mobile: (+91) 9555590180

Preface

A pediatric nurse has diversified roles in child health care. She acts as a counselor and has a pivotal role in establishing link between child's family on the one hand and the medical staff on the other. Therefore her approach, attitudes, communication and her bedside outlook related to child health care has to be oriented to the requirements of their own setup as well as hospital facilities. Due to penetration of modern technologies in the health care system and increasing burden on nurses they always search for ready reference, which is available with complete resources and new technologies.

The purpose of writing this book is to provide comprehensive, easy to understand procedures handbook. Extensive brain storming and comparison with standard reference books has been done to provide unambiguous materials to the student and faculties, which is also strictly in adherence with syllabus given by Indian Nursing Council. This book includes important guidelines so that standard performance can be evaluated by using standard checklist. This book will be a valuable weapon to all of them.

I do not claim any original contribution to the body of knowledge of pediatrics. But I tried my best to incorporate the latest information available and maintain standards in pediatric nursing.

I hope this book will not only help in improving the quality of training in pediatric nursing but also stimulate the nursing teachers into similar ventures.

I also earnestly invite suggestions and comments from the students and teachers about the book at my email-das.nyati@yahoo.co.in

I wish all the success in nursing career!

Niyati Das

Acknowledgements

First and foremost, this acknowledgement is to express my deep sense of gratitude to Almighty God for His abundant blessing and guidance to write this book.

It gives me great pleasure to acknowledge heartfelt thanks to my husband and family for their support.

It is my proud privilege to acknowledge my sincere thanks, humble regards and everlasting obligation to my professor Mrs Amrita Lenka, Principal, Kalinga Institute of Nursing Sciences for her constant guidance, support and motivation toward completing this book.

I also acknowledge my students for their interest to get this book, which inspired me to write.

My special thanks to Miss Purnima Sahoo. Assistant Professor, KINS for her untiring efforts in completing this book.

I acknowledge my teachers for their expertize and diligent guidance who really have rounded and polished my ideas in the touchstone of their experience and knowledge.

I take this opportunity to express my deep sense of gratitude to all experts from which I borrowed materials for ready references.

I acknowledge my deep sense of thanks to all nonteaching staffs for their support.

I acknowledge Mr Deepak Yadav, executive member of CBS Publishers whose effort and guidance helps me in the completion of this book.

I appreciate support of **Mr Satish Kumar Jain** (Chairman) and **Mr Varun Jain** (Managing Director), M/s CBS Publishers and Distributors Pvt Ltd. for their whole-hearted support in publication of this book. No amount of words can describe role, efforts, inputs and initiatives undertaken by **Mr Bhupesh Arora**, (Vice President-Publishing and Marketing, PGMEE and Nursing Division), for his endeavor toward the development of the book.

I thank Dr Mrinalini Bakshi (Sr Content Developer and Editor) for her editorial support and Ms Nitasha Arora (Project Manager), Ms Neetu Jindal (Asst. Production Manager), Mr Nitish K Dubey (Senior Editor) and all the production team members Mr Ashutosh Pathak, Mr Phool Kumar, Mr Bunty Kashyap, Mr Chaman Lal, Mr Prakash Gaur, Mr Deepak Kashyap, Ms Tahira Praveen, Ms Babita Verma, Mr Raju Sharma, Vikram Chaudhary, Manoj Chaudhary and Manoj Malakar for devoting laborious hours in designing and typesetting of this book. I convey thanks to all those who are associated with this book.

Contents

1

General Procedures

- Hand Washing
- Admission Procedure
- Checklist for Admission of Children
- Discharge Procedure

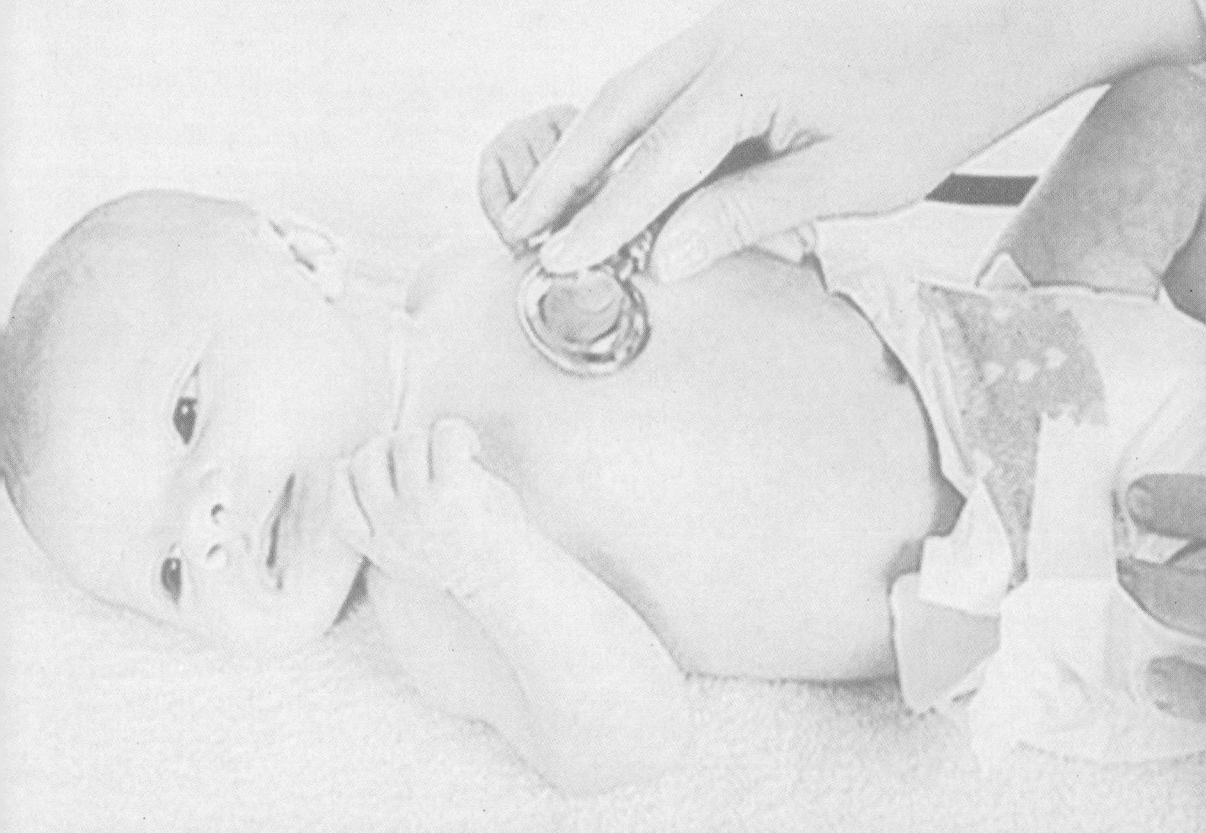

LEARNING OBJECTIVES

On completion of this chapter, the pediatric nurse will be able to perform the following activities:
- Demonstrate medical and surgical hand washing
- Practice personal protective equipment
- Define admission and types of admissions
- Understand the admission and discharge procedure
- Develop skills in admission and discharge of children
- Use checklist as an evaluation tool by teachers and students.

HAND WASHING

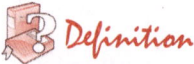 *Definition*

Hand washing is a process of mechanically removing the microorganisms from the hands and forearms with the use of soap and water.

- Articles needed
  - Soap in a soap dish
  - Nail brush
  - Hand towel

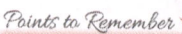 *Points to Remember*

- Remove jewellery from hands
- Finger nails should be short trimmed
- Fold sleeves approximately 2–3 inches above the elbows before starting the procedure.

Steps of Hand-Washing Technique

First of all, wet both hands and apply soap or liquid hand wash on them. Rub both hands. Perform the following steps as shown in Figures 1A to L.
- Rub palms together
- Rub the back of both hands one after another
- Interface fingers and rub the hands together
- Interlock fingers and rub the back of fingers of both hands
- Grasp the right hand's thumb inside the left hand's palm and rub it in a rotating manner and vice versa
- Knuckles fingertips on palm for both hands
- Rub both wrist in a rotating manner and rinse then thoroughly under running water and dry hands with a clean towel.

Hand hygiene should be performed in 5 instances: Before patient contact, before a procedure, after a procedure or body fluid exposure risk, after patient contact and after contact with patients surroundings, as per World Health Organization (WHO), 2006 Table 1 shows the checklist it for hand hygiene.

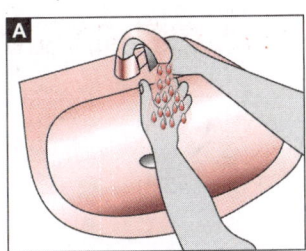

Wet hands with water

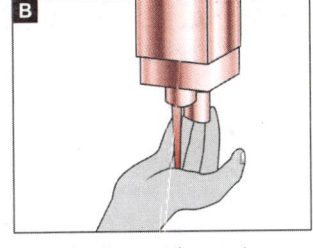

Apply enough soap to cover all hand surfaces

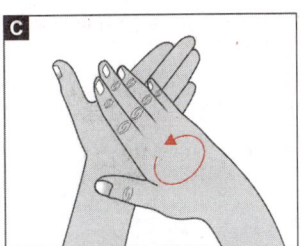

Rub hands palm to palm

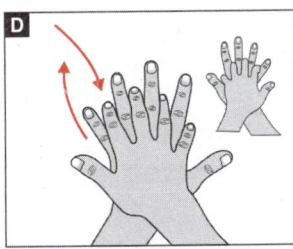

Right palm over left dorsum with interlaced fingers and vice versa

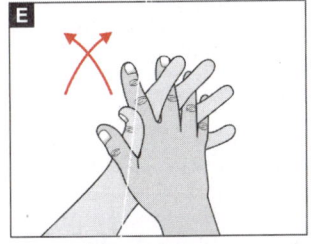

Palm to palm with fingers interlaced

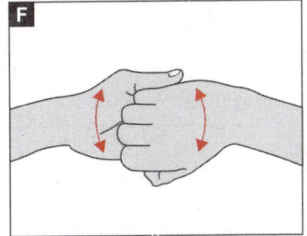

Backs of fingers to opposing palms with fingers interlocked

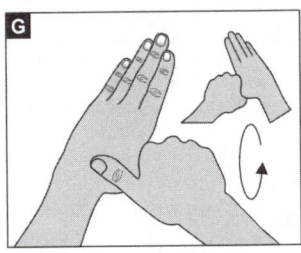

Rotational rubbing of left thumb clasped in right palm and vice versa

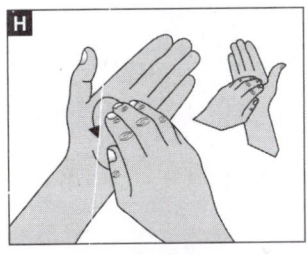

Rotational rubbing backwards and forwards with clasped fingers of right hand in left palm and vice versa

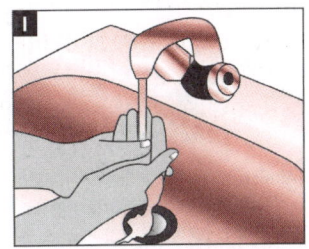

Rinse hands with water

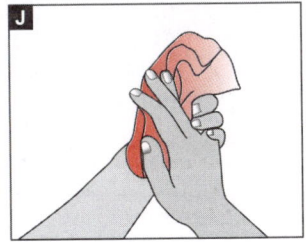

Dry throroughly with a towel

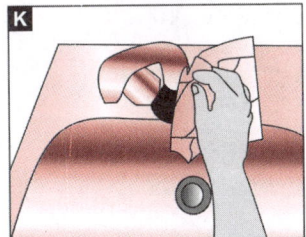

Use towel to turn off faucet

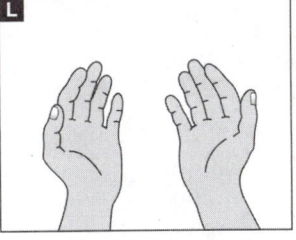

.. and your hands are safe

FIGS 1A to L: Hand washing technique

TABLE 1: Hand hygiene

Checklist for Hand Washing	Y	N
Remove rings, bracelets and watch		
Wet hands in clean running water. Apply soap		
Vigorously rub hands together in the following manner: • Palms, fingers and web spaces • Back of hands • Fingers and knuckles • Thumbs • Fingertips and creases • Wrist and forearm up to the elbow • Thoroughly rinse hands in clean running water. • Dry hands using a clean personal towel, paper towel, or allow to air dry.		

Score: Yes =1 and No = 0

Below 50%	Poor
50–60%	Average
61–70%	Good
71–80%	Very good
Above 80%	Excellent

ADMISSION PROCEDURE

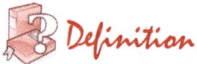 *Definition*

Admission is a process of allowing a patient to stay in the hospital for observation, investigation and treatment of the disease he or she is suffering from.

Articles Needed

- Admission bed or open bed
- Bed crib, warmer or bassinet and isollete
- Blankets, linens, bath towel and wash clothes
- Toiletry items
- A jar with drinking water and glass
- Diaper and wipe
- Bedpan and urinal
- Identification band for the child
- Scissors
- Measuring tape
- Weighing machine
- Vital signs tray
- Pulse oximeter
- Patient admission documentation forms

Types of Admission

The admission of a patient to a hospital can be of two types:

- **Routine Admission:** It means patient are admitted for investigation, planned treatment and surgeries, e.g. patient with diabetes, chronic appendicitis, hernia, cirrhosis of liver, chronic renal failure, etc.
- **Emergency Admission:** This type of admission means that patient's are admitted in serious condition to the casualty or emergency department so that immediate treatment is initiated to save the life of patient's e.g. patient with heart attack, accident, labor pain, poisoning, shock, etc.

The admission is done in following two departments:

I. **Outpatient Department:** It is also known as OPD

   Following procedures are followed in OPD

   - **Reception of patient:** First impression is likely very important and not easily erased, it is important for patient and his family members to get attention. In emergency condition, no time should be wasted to initiate the treatment. The manner in which the nurse and physician receive and treat the patient is after all most important aspect of reception and admission to the hospital.

   - **Recording of social and medical data:** Record section is responsible for identification of patient. It questions the patient or his/her family members to get the name, age, sex, address, religion, income, marital status, phosne number, etc. Necessary data is supplied by family and friends at first opportunity. This can be obtained by appropriate questioning of the patient.

   - **Medical examination:** A detailed social and medical history of patient is taken by the physician and is recorded.

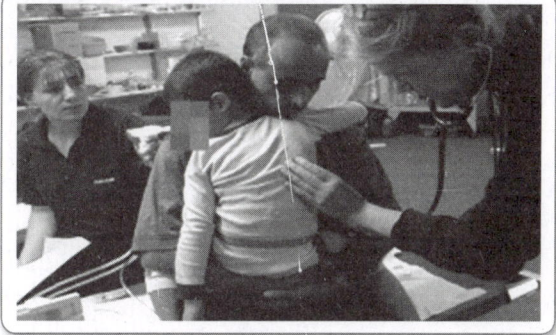

FIG. 2: Physical examination of child

   The patient's temperature, pulse, blood pressure, etc. are recorded. In this procedure head to toe examination is done. The investigations like X-ray, lab tests, CT scan, etc. are done for final diagnosis of a disease.

II. **Inpatient department:** Those who are suffering from mild ailments are sent home with necessary treatment in OPD. Those with serious aliments are admitted to the hospital for further investigations and treatment.

   - **Transporting patient from OPD to IPD:** Patients with minor ailments are allowed to walk by nurse or attendants. Wheel chairs should be available for those who are suffering form some serious ailments, weak or are unable to walk or in emergency case nurse should carry the patient in the ambulance to their respective wards.

Box 1

TIPS FOR ADMITTING THE CHILD TO IPD

- Reception of the child.
- Preliminary observation of child.
- Helping the child to occupy his bed.
- Care of the clothing and valuables.
- Orient the parents and child.
- Building rapport with child and parent.
- Eliciting the case- history.
- Carrying out the physician orders.
- Documentation, report to ward sister.

- **Reception of patient by ward sister:** Ward sister admitting patient should introduce herself and should greet patient and his relatives with full respect (Fig. 3).
- If the patient is too sick, she should put him/her to bed immediately.
- **Preliminary observation of the patient:** The patient's general facial expression will tell not only his emotional reaction but also presence of pain.
- **Helping the patient to occupy his bed:** A close bed is converted to an open bed on admission of patient. If the patient is unconscious then the nurse should help him/her to occupy the bed.

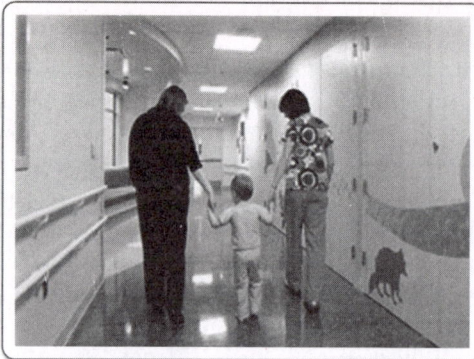

FIG. 3: Reception of patient in inpatient department by ward sister

- **Care of valuable things and clothing:** While an undressing the patient, ensured it should be that his/her dirty clothes should be sent home with relatives for washing and clean cloths should be kept safely for daily use. In absence of relatives these should be numbered and labeled and kept in store until that is handled over to relatives. In case of communicable disease, clothing should be disinfected in an appropriate manner.

Box 2

Nurse's Responsibility in Admission Procedure
- Establish nurse patient relationship mainly with parents and family
- Introduce yourself and smile with child
- Orient to child and parents about the hospital unit
- Explain the child and family members about the hospital policy and regulation
- Ask the family and child what names they prefer to be called by
- Maintain eye contact at the appropriate level
- Obtain information about the child's history, routines and reason for admission
- Assess base line vital signs, height and weight and perform physical assessment

CHECKLIST FOR ADMISSION OF CHILDREN

Task	YES	NO
Getting ready with the following articles:		
• Admission bed or open bed		
• Bed crib, warmer or bassinet, isollete		
• Blankets, linens, bath towel, wash clothes		
• Toiletry items		
• A jar with drinking water and glass		
• Diaper and wipe		
• Bed pan, urinal		
• Identification band for child		
• Scissors		
• Measuring tape		
• Weighing machine		
• Vital signs tray		
• Pulse oximeter		
• Patient admission documentation forms		

Yes-1, no-0

Below 50%	Poor
50–60%	Average
61–70%	Good
71–80%	Very good
Above 80%	Excellent

DISCHARGE PROCEDURE

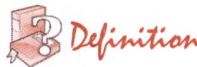 Definition

When a patient is stable after receiving the treatment, he/she gets permission on to leave the hospital. This is known as discharge.

Preparation of the Patient for Discharge

- **Rehabilitation of the patient:** Rehabilitation means treatment and training of the patient to the end that he may attain his maximal potential for normal living physically, psychologically and socially. It begins when a patient contacts the health care team for the first time.
- Planning for patient's discharge:
  - A day has to be fixed for termination of care and the date has to be informed his/her family members. Relatives have to follow hospital instructions without hurry and bring the clothing for the patient.
  - After this patient should be aware about the time and dose of the medicines which he has to continue at home or about some procedure advised to continue at home after discharge.
  - The patient should be demonstrated and made familiar with type of diet he has to continue at home.
  - At last nurse has to watch for reaction of patient about his discharge. Most patients are happy when their physician tells them that they can leave the hospital.

Procedure

- No patient should be discharged without the doctor's order. The physician writes on the patient's chart when the patient is to be discharged. Instructions regarding further care, medication, treatment, follow-up etc. should be clearly written and interpreted to the patient and his family members.
- Patient's personal belongings such as clothing, money and other valuable things which were entrusted to the hospital at the time of admission should be checked and returned to him.
- Any of hospital's property that was given to patient for his/her use in hospital should be checked and received back before he leaves.
- Before patient leaves the hospital, the nurse should confirm whether he has paid all the hospital bills.
- The patient should be made ready by giving a proper bath, combing the hair and dressed neatly in his/her clothes.
- If the patient is unable or not allowed to walk nurse should either provide a wheel chair or a stretcher during transfer for safely.

- The dietary department should be informed of the patient's discharge.
- If any patient leaves the hospital against medical advice, he should be asked to sign a release form where it should be mentioned that patient is leaving against advice of doctor. Neither doctor nor hospital can be held responsible for any effect happening after his departure.
- Nurse should see the charts are completed and sent to the office for the record section to be filled.

Care of Patient's Unit after Discharge of a Patient

- After discharge of a patient, room is cleaned and purified.
- Windows and doors are opened.
- Furniture and light shades are washed and cleaned.
- Articles used by patient should be taken to utility room, washed and sterilized before use by another patient.
  - Used linen are sent to laundry and mattress, pillows and blankets should be exposed to sunlight and a close bed should be made. If room is used for any patient suffering from communicable disease it should be fumigated with articles.

Box 3

STEPS-PREPARATION OF CHILD FOR DISCHARGE
- Rehabilitation of the patient
- Planning for the patient's discharge
- Discharge procedure
- Care of the child's unit after discharge
- Advice for follow up

2

Health Assessment of Children

- ⊃ Pediatric History Taking
- ⊃ Immunization History
- ⊃ Vital Signs

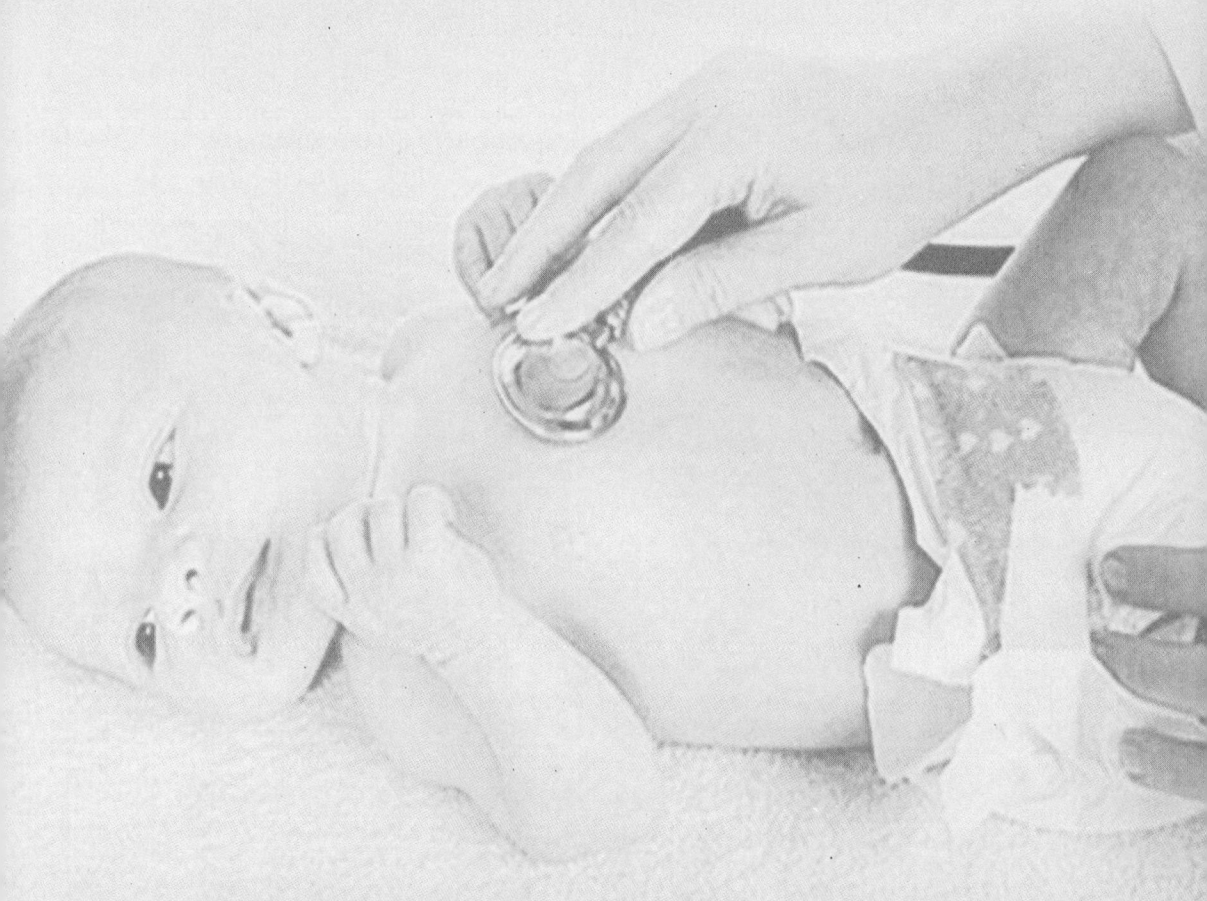

LEARNING OBJECTIVES

On completion of this chapter, the pediatric nurse will be able to perform the following activities:
- Elicit the case history
- Enlist the process of history taking
- Use checklist for pediatric history taking

PEDIATRIC HISTORY TAKING

INTRODUCTION

The history of a child is obtained to establish a relationship with the child and the family. In history collection, focus should be on a specific topic depending on the child's stages of growth such as infant, toddler, school age and adolescence.

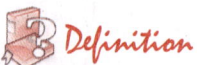 *Definition*

Pediatric history taking is a proper collection of information regarding a child from the parents, relatives or by child itself (if able to talk) for purposeful evaluation aspects.

PURPOSE OF HISTORY TAKING

- To establish and maintain a good relationship with the child and his/her family members
- To collect the data for the diagnosis and treatment
- To clear the doubts of parents regarding the child's health, treatment plan or any other concepts
- To prepare an effective plan of care to fulfill the needs of the child.

 *Points to Remember*

General Instructions for a Nurse
- Always use local/appropriate language for collecting the information
- Always ask the relevant questions only and follow a friendly approach
- Ask the questions according to the understanding level of the child
- Allow the family members to express the real information. Do not force them
- All the information should be recorded in a file immediately
- Maintain a good inter-personal relationship with the family.

Box 1

Always ask to parents 'BIFIDA'
- B-Birth details and problems
- I-Immunization history
- F-Feeding problems
- I-Infection and exposure detail
- D-Developmental history
- A-Allergic reaction

Box 2

The life-threatening events: 'THEMISFITS' assessment tool:

- T-Trauma
- H-Heart disease or hypovolemia
- E-Electrolyte disturbance
- M-Metabolic disturbance
- I-Inborn errors of metabolism
- S-Sepsis
- F-Formula dilution or over concentration
- I-Intestinal catastrophe
- T-Toxins
- S-Seizures or CNS abnormalities

Box 3

Protocol of History Collection
- Patient's profile
- Presenting complaints
- History of present illness
- Past history
- Family history and family tree
- Socioeconomic status of the family
- Personal history
- Birth history
- Feeding history
- Immunization
- Physical examination
- Developmental history
- Drug history

PATIENT'S PROFILE

- Name of the patient
- Chronological age (DOB)
- Developmental stage
- Sex
- Address of the patient
- Date of admission

Presenting Complaints

- Use parent's own word and follow chronological order
- Patient tells about the symptoms such as
  - My head is hurting—Headache
  - I cannot feel my foot—Loss of sensation in foot

Chronological Order

- Site—Where is the pain?
- Onset—When did the pain start?
- Character—What was the pain like?
- Quality—Severity of the pain
- Variation—Seasonal or diurnal
- Associated symptoms

HISTORY OF PRESENT ILLNESS

More attention should be paid on the onset of illness, complete interval history, the status and the reason for admission. The following data should be collected:

- A. Enquire about the last time patient was entirely well
- B. Systemic enquiry
- General—Weight loss, appetite
- CVS—Shortness of breath, cyanotic spells, cyanosis, edema
- Respiratory system—Sore throat, earache, cough, wheeze
- GI system—Abdominal pain, vomiting, jaundice
- CNS—Fits, syncope, visual problem, numbness
- Genitourinary system—Dysuria, nocturnal incontinence, hematuria
- Rheumatic system—Limb swelling, dry mouth, hair loss, skin rash.

HISTORY OF MOTHER DURING AND AFTER PREGNANCY

- Antenatal history (History of pregnancy)
- Hypertension and nutritional status
- Illness during pregnancy
- Quality of fetal movement
- X-ray and other investigational reports of each trimester
- Drugs taken during gestation
- Post-obstetric history

NATAL HISTORY (HISTORY OF DELIVERY)

- Place of delivery
- Conducted by
- Sterilization technique
- Gestation time
- Labor time
- Presentation and type of delivery
- Sedation used during labor
- Complications (if any)
- Expected date of delivery and the approximate duration of pregnancy.

POSTNATAL HISTORY

- Duration of hospitalization of mother and infant
- Any problem with baby's feeding and breathing
- Nature of first cry
- Birth weight
- Birth injury
- Any other problems
- Bowel movements

FEEDING HISTORY

- This is significant mainly in children above 2 years of age as shown in Figure 1.
- Onset of feeding
- Type of feed
- Supplement
- Weaning
- Current diet or change of diet during illness
- Age of weaning
- Pattern of weight gain
- Current diet

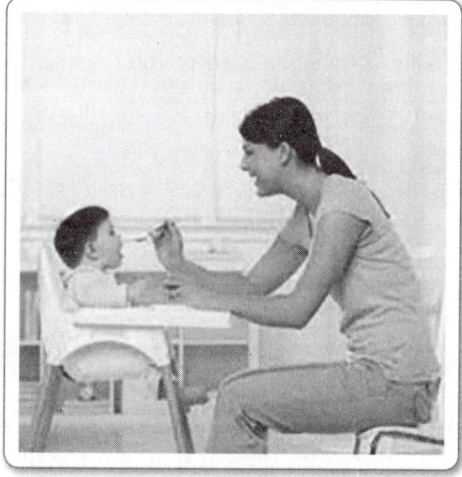

FIG. 1: Feeding the child

FAMILY HISTORY

- Age of mother and father? How long are they married?
- Consanguinity
- Parents health
- Sibling—number, age and sex
- Illness
- Any death
- Stillbirth or miscarriage
- Grandparents' health (Fig. 2)

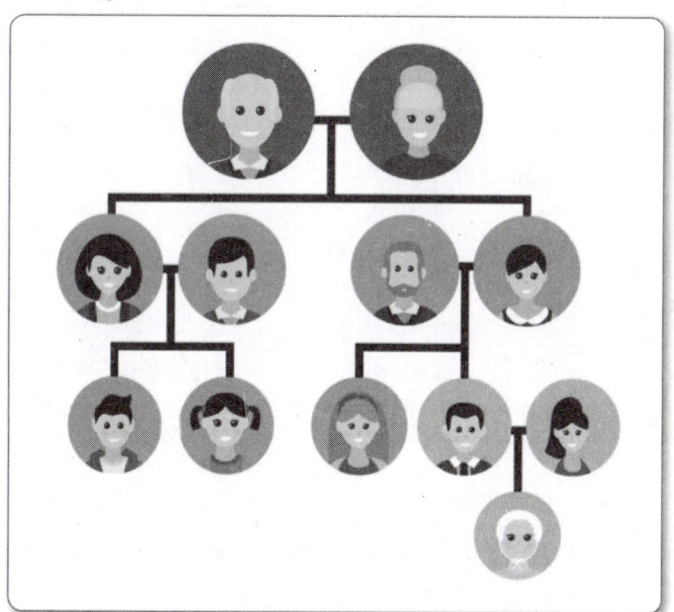

FIG. 2: Family tree showing how the health of grandparents is connected to the health of the child

DEVELOPMENTAL HISTORY

Detailed developmental screening should be conducted. Age-appropriate special milestones are to be asked and noted.

HABITS

Age-appropriate habits and their variations are asked such as the eating, sleeping and toilet habits of the child.

TABLE 1: Checklist for pediatric history taking

Task	Y	N
Getting ready with the following prerequisites: Room with well-lighted, comfortable, quiet and decorated with play materials, chairs and examination table, computer, paper and pen to record the history		
Patient's profile		
Presenting complaints		
History of present illness		
Past history		
Family history and family tree		
Socioeconomic status of the family		
Personal history, birth history, feeding pattern		
Immunization history, growth and development assessment		
Documentation, report to ward sister		

Score: Yes = 1 and No = 0. Below 50%; poor

50–60%	Average
61–70%	Good
71–80%	Very good
Above 80%	Excellent

IMMUNIZATION HISTORY

IMMUNIZATION SCHEDULE STATUS

This information is useful to guide the diagnosis and ensures holistic management of the child.

TABLE 2: Immunization schedule (IAP latest)

Age	Vaccines	Note
Birth	BCG	
	OPV zero	
	Hepatitis B-1	
6 weeks	OPV-1 + IPV-1/OPV-1	OPV alone if IPV cannot be given
	DTPw-1/DTPa-1	
	Hepatitis B-2	
	Hib-1	
10 weeks	OPV-2 + IPV-2/OPV-2	OPV alone if IPV cannot be given
	DTPw-2/DTPa-2	
	Hib-2	
14 weeks	OPV-3 + IPV-3/OPV-3	OPV alone if IPV cannot be given
	DTPw-3/DTPa-3	
	Hepatitis B-3	Third dose of hepatitis B can be given at 6 months of age
	Hib-3	
9 months	Measles	
15–18 months	OPV-4 + IPV-B1/OPV-4	OPV alone if IPV cannot be given
	DTPw booster-1 or DTPa booster-1	
	Hib booster	
	MMR-1	
2 years	Typhoid	Revaccination every 3–4 years
5 years	OPV-5	
	DTPw booster-2 or DTPa booster-2	
	MMR-2	The second dose of MMR vaccine can be given at any time 8 weeks after the first dose
10 years	Tdap	
	HPV	Only girls, three doses at 0, 1–2 and 6 months
	Vaccines that can be given after discussion with parents	
More than 6 weeks	Pneumococcal conjugate	3 primary doses at 6, 10 and 14 weeks, followed by a booster at 15–18 months
More than 6 weeks	Rotavirus vaccines	2/3 doses (depending on brand) at 4–8 weeks interval
After 15 months	Varicella	Age less than 13 years: One dose age more than 13 years: 2 doses at 4–8 weeks interval
After 18 months	Hepatitis A	2 doses at 6–12 months interval

TABLE 3: National immunization schedule in India 2017

Vaccine	Prevents	Minimum age for dose 1	Interval between dose 1 and 2	Interval between dose 2 and 3	Interval between dose 3 and 4	Interval between dose 4 and 5
BCG	TB and bladder cancer	Birth				
Hep B	Hepatitis B	Birth	4 weeks	8 weeks		
Poliovirus	Polio	Birth	4 weeks	4 weeks		
DTP	Diphtheria, tetanus and pertussis	6 weeks	4 weeks	4 weeks	6 months (booster 1)	3 years (booster 2)
Hib	Infections caused by bacteria	6 weeks	4 weeks	4 weeks	6 months (booster 1)	
PCV	Pneumonia	6 weeks	4 weeks	4 weeks	6 months (booster 1)	
RV	Severe diarrheal disease	6 weeks	4 weeks	4 weeks		
Typhoid	Typhoid fever, diarrhea	9 months	15 months (booster 1)			
MMR	Measles, mumps and rubella	9 months	6 months			
Varicella	Chickenpox	1 year	3 months			
Hep A	Liver disease	1 year	6 months			
Tdap	Diphtheria, tetanus and pertussis	7 years				
HPV	Some cancers and warts	9 years	• For child aged 9–14 years: 6 months • For child aged 15 or more: 1 month	For child aged 15 or more: 5 months		

ADMINISTRATION OF VACCINES

Steps of Administering the Vaccines

- Keep necessary items ready: Vaccine carrier, hub cutter, cotton, 0.5 mL syringe, immunization card
- Check the expiry date on the vaccine vial to make sure the vaccine is in usable stage
- Shake the vial to observe freezing or floccules or particulate matter. Discard the vial if any of these are present
- Position the child on the mother's lap in such a way that the child's head rests on mother's right arm with left arm of the child placed at the back of mother and mother's right hand holds child's right hand. With the left hand, the mother holds the child's both legs

- Open a fresh 0.5 mL AD syringe and throw syringe wrapper and cap in a black bag. Load the vaccine into syringe
- Expel excess air from the syringe by tapping it and make sure that the syringe has exactly 0.5 ml of vaccine
- Put finger and thumb of the left hand on either side of the injection site (right anterolateral thigh)
- Stretch the skin flat between finger and thumb
- Hold the syringe like a pen in the right hand and push the needle straight down at 90 degrees
- Press the top of the plunger with the thumb to inject the vaccine
- Withdraw the needle and press the site of injection with a dry cotton swab
- Cut the needle with a hub cutter and put the plastic part of a syringe into red bag
- Document the immunization card and provide four key messages about immunization
- Which vaccine should be given and which disease does the vaccine protect against?
  - When to come for the next vaccination?
  - Effects of immunization such as localized pain, redness, swelling at injection site, injection site nodule and low-grade fever
  - How to manage the same by giving paracetamol for fever, cold cloth at injection site for local reaction
- Keep immunization card safe and bring it on the next visit.

Administration of BCG Vaccine

- Keep the necessary items ready, vaccine carrier with BCG vaccine and diluent (normal saline), 5 mL mixing syringe, BCG syringe (0.1 mL AD syringe), cotton, hub cutter and immunization card

Checks

- Whether it is the right vaccine and diluent
- The vaccine has not passed its expiry date and VVM is in usable stage
- Open an ampoule of diluent and draw 1 mL of diluent into a fresh sterile mixing syringe
- Insert the mixing needle into vial of vaccine and empty the diluent in it and withdraw the syringe
- Cut the hub of the mixing syringe with a hub cutter, discard the plastic part of the syringe in a red bag
- Mix the vaccine and diluent by gently shaking the vial with one hand. Write the time and date of reconstitution on the label
- Ask the parent to take child on her lap, and hold the child firmly. Baby's head rests on mother's left arm. Baby's left arm and legs are controlled by the mother's right arm and hand
- Open a fresh 0.1 mL AD syringe and throw syringe wrapper and cap in a black bag. Load the BCG syringe with reconstituted BCG vaccine with a dose of 0.05 mL
- Position the left hand under child's left arm and gently pull the skin under the arm to stretch the skin at injection site
- Hold the syringe in the right hand, with the bevel of the needle facing up. Lay the syringe and needle almost flat (at an angle of 15°) along the child's arm
- Put the left thumb over needle end of the syringe (not on the needle) to hold it in position
- Hold the plunger between the index and the middle finger of the right hand and press the plunger with the right thumb
- Inject vaccine and withdraw the needle
- Look for clear, flat-topped swelling on the skin (bleb)
- Cut the hub of the syringe with a hub cutter and put the plastic part in a red bag

- Document the immunization card and provide four key messages about immunization
  - Which vaccine should be given and which disease does the vaccine protect against?
  - When to come for the next vaccination?
  - Effects and side effects of immunization and how to manage the same: After 2–3 weeks a papule develops, which increases slowly in size up to 5 weeks (4–8 mm). It will then subside and break into a shallow ulcer; healing will occur in 4–8 weeks, following a permanent scar
- Keep immunization card safe and bring it on the next visit

VITAL SIGNS

Vital signs are a measurement of four essential components:
- Blood pressure
- Heart rate
- Respiratory rate
- Temperature

The normal values of vital signs vary with the age of the child (Table 4). Some can be lower than the adults while others can be higher. The average vital signs for the different age groups of children are mentioned below:

TABLE 4: Normal values of vital signs with the age of the child

• Infants	
Vital signs	**Normal values**
Heart rate	
• Newborn to 1 month	85–190 beats/minute
• 1 month to 1 year	90–180 beats/minute
Respiratory rate	30–60 per minute
Temperature	98.6° Fahrenheit
Blood pressure	
• Newborn to 1 month	67–84 mm Hg/31–45 mm Hg
• 1 month to 1 year	72–104 mm Hg/37–56 mm Hg
• Toddler (1 to 2 years old)	
Vital signs	**Normal values**
Heart Rate	98–140 beats/minute
Respiratory rate	22–37 per minute
Blood pressure	86–106 mm Hg/42–63 mm Hg
Temperature	98.6° Fahrenheit
• Preschooler (3 to 5 years old)	
Vital sign	**Normal values**
Heart rate	80–120 beats/minute
Respiratory rate	20–28 per minute
Blood Pressure	89–112 mm Hg/46–72 mm Hg
Temperature	98.6° Fahrenheit

Contd...

• School going child (6 to 11 years old)	
Vital signs	**Normal values**
Heart rate	75–118 beats/minute
Respiratory rate	18–25 per minute
Blood pressure	97–120 mm Hg/57–80 mm Hg
Temperature	98.6° Fahrenheit
• Adolescent (12 years and above)	
Vital signs	**Normal values**
Heart Rate	60–100 beats/minute
Respiratory rate	12–20 per minute
Blood pressure	110–131 mm Hg/64–83 mm Hg
Temperature	98.6° Fahrenheit

CHECKING THE TEMPERATURE

Temperature can be assessed with the help of a thermometer.

Steps of Temperature Assessment

Oral Route (Older Children)

- Clean the thermometer and switch it on.
- Keep thermometer under the tongue on the side of the frenulum.
- Once the beep is heard, take out the thermometer and note the reading.

Axillary Route

This is the most preferred method in small children.

- Clean the thermometer and the axilla. The axilla should be dry.
- After turning on the thermometer, it should be placed in the center of axilla and the arm should be held tightly across the chest to avoid displacement of thermometer.
- Once the beep is heard, remove the thermometer and note the reading.

Monitoring the Respiration

The respiratory rate can be assessed in the following ways:

- Help the patient to position comfortably with hands across his/her chest
- Avoid moving the hand and patient's arm and count the number of breaths in one miute
- Complete rise and fall of chest should be counted as 1
- Note the number of breaths along with the character of respiration like the regularity, ease, etc.

3

Assessment of Physical Growth of Children

- Weight
- Height
- Head Circumference
- Chest Circumference
- Mid-Arm Circumference

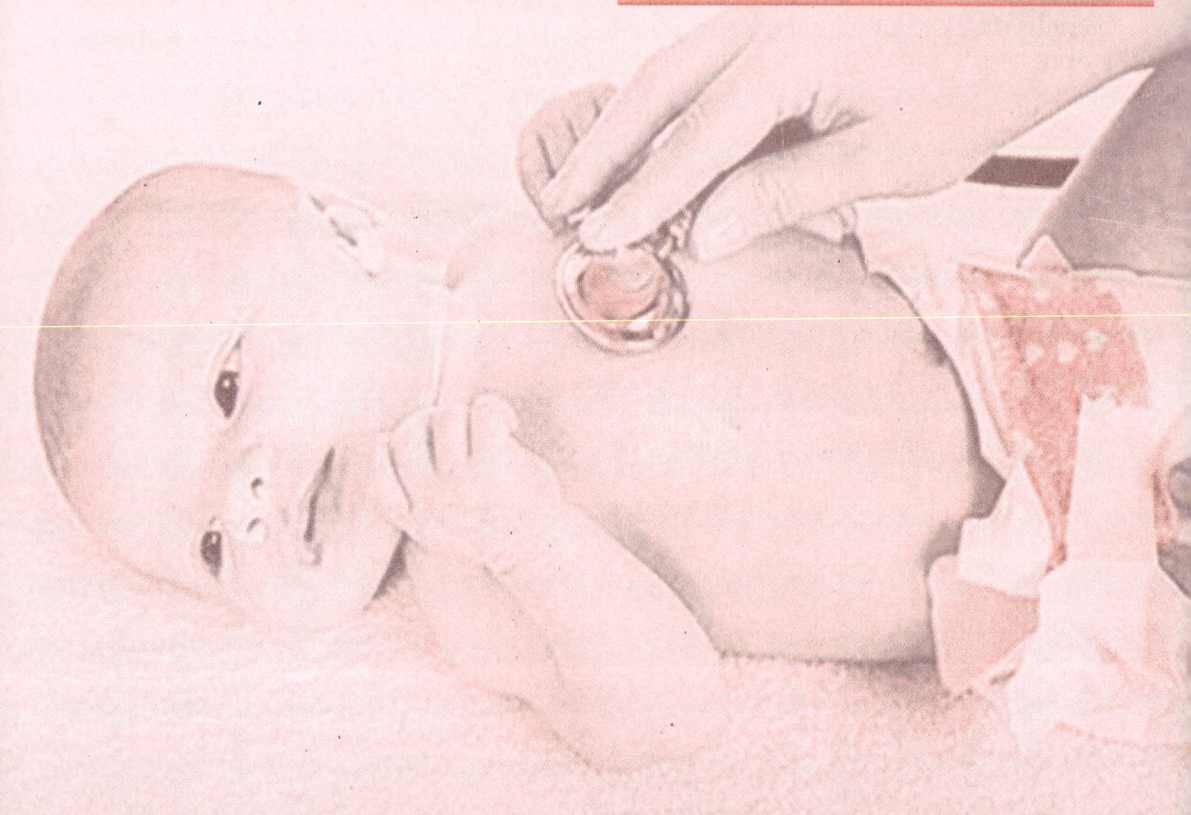

LEARNING OBJECTIVES

On completion of this chapter, the pediatric nurse will be able to perform the following activities:
- Identify the anthropometric measurement parameters in detail
- Develop skills in measuring these parameters
- Compare with standard values of parameters used for of children

INTRODUCTION

The measurement of various anthropometric data is essential for assessing the growth and nutritional status of the child.

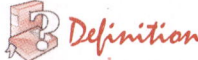 Definition

Anthropometric measurement means measuring the height, weight, head, chest and mid-arm circumference of the child.

Purposes

- To calculate the nutritional requirements
- To assess the degree of malnutrition
- To monitor the growth
- To calculate the dosages of medication.

Articles Needed

- Weighing scale appropriate for the child's age (Conventional beam balance scale, hanging scale, ground scale and electronic weighing machine)
- Disposable papers for covering the scale
- Infantometer/height scale fixed against the wall
- Scale or pointer
- Pen and paper
- Measuring tape and shakir tape.

WEIGHT

- The newborn loses up to 10% of its weight during the 1st week, but regains it in the next few days.
- The average birthweight of newborn is 2.5 kg and it increases at the rate of 500 to 600 g per month during first 6 months.
- Weight is recorded on a weighing scale which should be frequently checked with standards weights. Zero error must be adjusted before weighing.
- The infant is weighed on an infant scale; the older child is weighed on an upright platform scale.

Box 1

According to Welch's formula:

Weight:
- At birth: 2.5–3 kg
- 2–12 months: Age in month + 9/2
- 1–6 years: Age in years × 2 + 8
- 7–12 years: Age in years × 7–5/2

Box 2

According to Ballpark
- Average birthweight: 2.5–3 kg
- Double the birth by 5 months: 5–6 kg
- Triple the birthweight by one year: 7.5–9 kg

Procedure (Fig. 1)

- Place the weighing scale on a flat and stable surface
- Check whether the pan is centrally placed
- Check whether the pan is free to move
- Place towel/autoclaved paper on the pan
- Adjust the setting to "0"
- Undress the baby and place the baby on the weighing machine
- The baby needs to be placed centrally on the pan
- Pacify the baby if he/she is vigorous
- Record the reading in the register
- Inform the mother about the baby's weight
- Remove the baby from the pan and dress the baby quickly
- Give the baby to the mother
- Clean the pan if it is soiled.

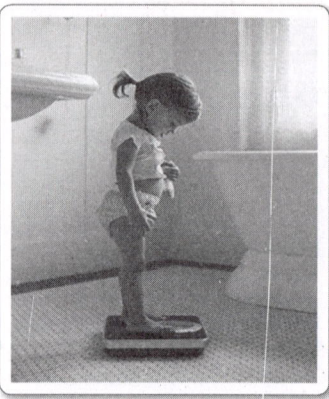

FIG. 1: Weight measurement of a child

HEIGHT (FIG. 2)

- Height is ideally measured using Holtain stadiometer.
- The child should stand against a wall with his/ her bare feet touching against the scale; ideally heels, buttock, upper back and occiput should touch the wall and the child should be looking straight ahead.

Box 3

Normal increase in height of children	
Age	**Height**
At birth	50 cm
6 months	+12 cm
1 year	75 cm
2 years	85 cm
2–5 years	6–8 cm/year
5 years and above	5 cm/year

- A measurement ruler is used to obtain length or height.
- Until the child can stand steadily, generally before the age of 5 years, the height is taken as length while the child is lying on a firm table.

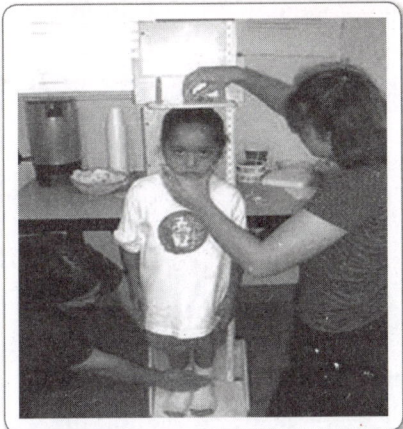

FIG. 2: Measuring height

Box 4

According to Welch's formula:
Expected height or normal children
At birth, baby's height is 50 cm (20 inch)
Average height is 48–52 cm (18–22 inch)
At 1 year = 75 cm/30 inches
2–12 years:
Age in years × 6 + 77 cm
Age in years × 2 + 30 (inches)

HEAD CIRCUMFERENCE (FIG. 3)

- Head circumference is measured with a nonstretchable tape passing through the maximum point of the external area of the head
- At birth, it is approximately 33–35 cm and increases at the rate of 1.5 cm per month during first 6 months.
- It varies from 32 cm to 35 cm at birth; from 43 cm to 46 cm at 1 year; and from 48 cm to 51 cm at 5 years.
- The adult head size is reached between 5 years and 6 years of age.

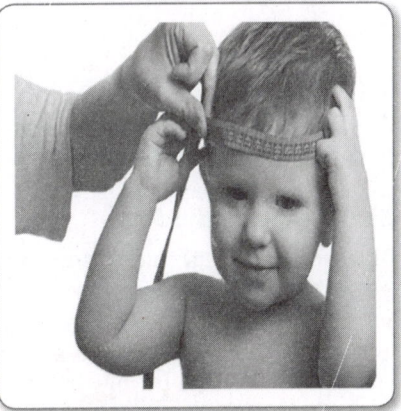

FIG. 3: Measurement of head circumference

Box 5

Height for age	Growth velocity
Till 3 months	2 cm/month
3 months–1 year	2 cm/3 months
1–3 years	1 cm/6 months
3–5 years	1 cm/year

CHEST CIRCUMFERENCE (FIG. 4)

- During mild respiration, the circumference of the chest is measured at the level of the nipple line.
- The measuring tape is placed at right angles to the vertebral column.
- The abdomen is measured up to 3 years of age in children with chronic intestinal problem.
- The chest circumference of the infant is lesser than the head circumference by about 2.5 cm and the two become equal by 1 year, after which the chest circumference exceeds the head circumference
- It is about 31–33 cm.

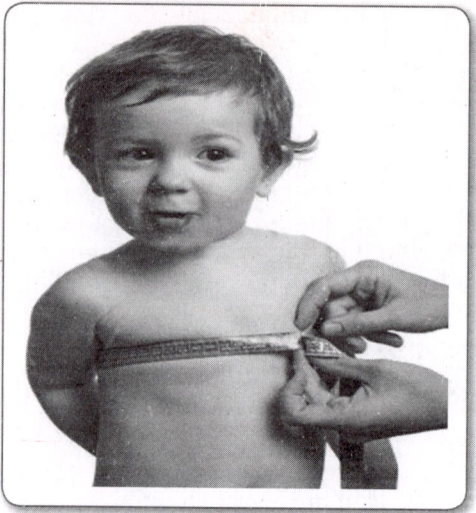

FIG. 4: Measurement of chest circumference

MILD-ARM CIRCUMFERENCE

- It is useful to detect malnutrition in young children (1–4 years).
- Values > 13.5 cm may be considered normal, while values < 12.5 cm indicate significant wasting of muscles and undernutrition.

Shakir Tape Method

This special tape has colored zones: Red, yellow, green, corresponding to:

- < 12.5 cm (wasted)
- 12.5–13.5 cm (border line) and
- Over 13.5 cm (normal) mid-arm circumference

ARM SPAN

- It is the distance between the tips of the middle fingers with both arms held mid apart, i.e. spread apart.
- Normally, in young children, arm span is 1–2 cm less than the length or height.
- It equals the height at 10 years and after 10 years it is 1–2 cm more than the height.
- An increased arm span is seen in Marfan's syndrome and homocystinuria.

ABDOMEN

- The measurement is made on a recumbent infant at the level of umbilicus with the measuring tape at right angles to the vertebral column. The abdomen of children is measured up to 3 years of age in children with chronic intestinal problem.
- At birth, an abdominal circumference is 32 cm (12.5 inch).
- The average abdominal circumference is 31–33 cm.

4

Physical Examination and Assessment

- ➲ Head to Toe Examination
- ➲ Neurological Assessment
- ➲ Developmental Assessment

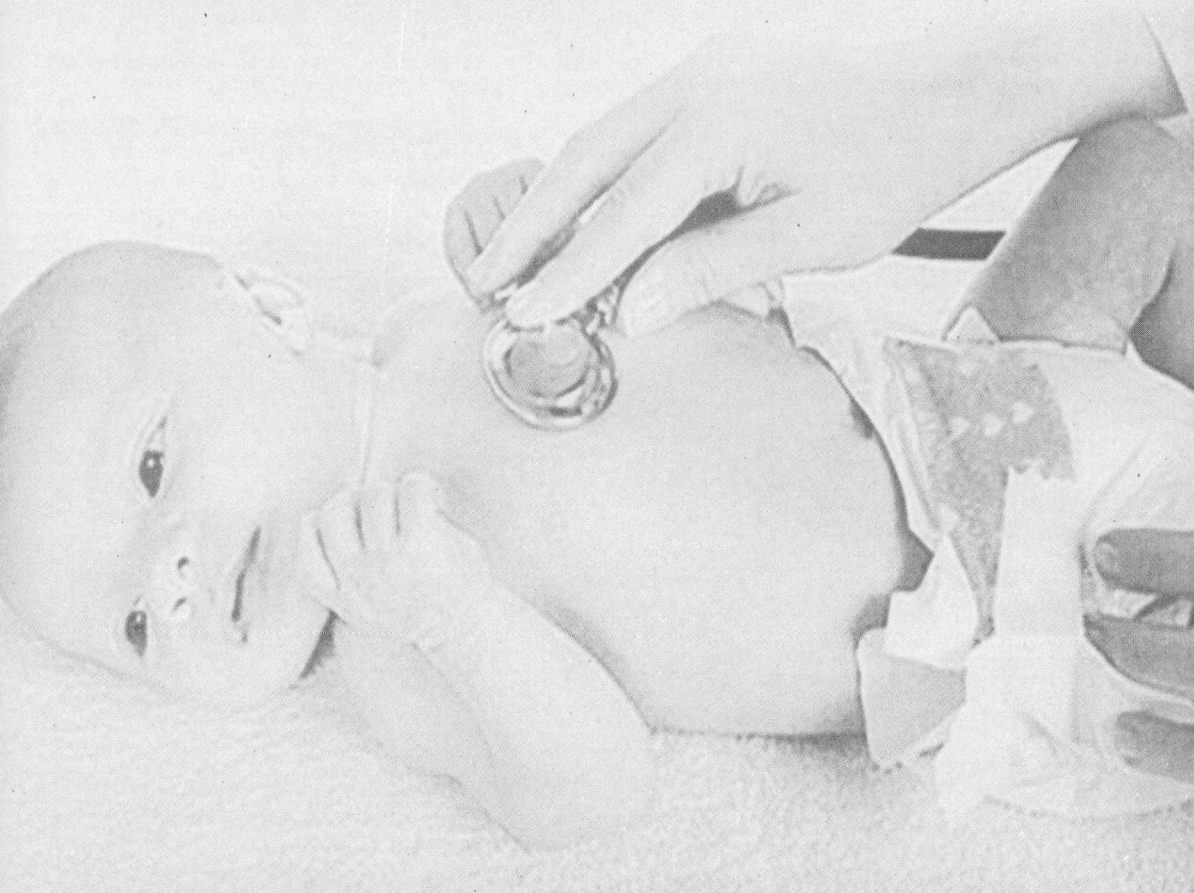

LEARNING OBJECTIVES

On completion of this chapter, the pediatric nurse will be able to do the following:
- Comprehend the purposes of a physical examination.
- Describe the techniques applied during a physical examination.
- Define development
- Explain purpose of developmental assessment
- Develop skills in assessment of development
- Apply the methods of developmental assessment
- Detect delay in development and treatment

HEAD TO TOE EXAMINATION

INTRODUCTION

Physical examination and health assessment is the most important part for correct diagnosis.

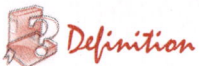 *Definition*

It is the systematic collection of objective information that is directly observed or is elicited through examination technique.

PURPOSE

- To understand physical and mental well-being
- To detect disease
- To determine the cause and extent of disease
- To determine the nature of treatment technique.

GENERAL PRINCIPLES

- Establish the order of data collection according to the patient's need
- If the parents have come in with more than one child, engage them in supervising the other child so that you can have some time with the patient alone
- The safest place for a young child is on the parent's knee; privacy may not be possible because of the presence of other children
- Develop good rapport with young children
- Explain to the school-going children about the procedure.

Approach to the Patient

- Begin the examination with the patient on parent's knee
- Evaluate the chest properly; listen 10 heartbeats when the child is not screaming
- The part of examination should be exposed
- Remember to examine everything may or (may not in systemic approach)
- Gradually remove the patient's cloths and carefully observe.
- Use of cold stethoscope approach may result in a frightened and screaming child, so warm the stethoscope before bringing it in contact with the child's skin.
- Show the child the procedure by demonstrating on parents.

Articles Needed

Glucometer (Fig. 1A)
- Thermometer (Fig. 1B)
- Stethoscope
- Tuning fork (Fig. 1C)
- Ophthalmoscope (Fig. 1D)
- Disposable gloves (Fig. 1F)
- Cotton applicator stick

- Tongue depressor
- Lubricant
- Reflex hammer
- Flashlight
- Knee hammer
- Torch (Fig. 1E)

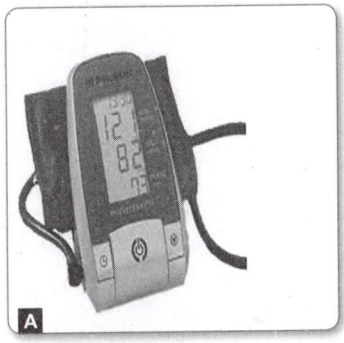 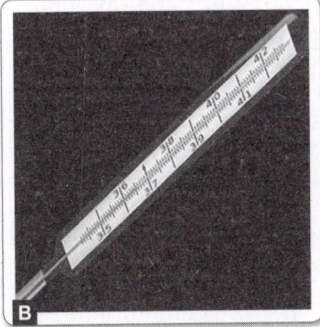 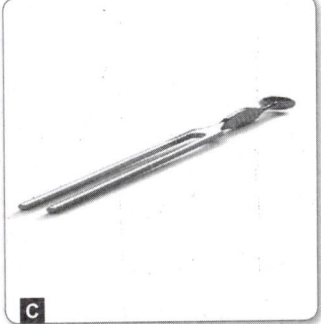

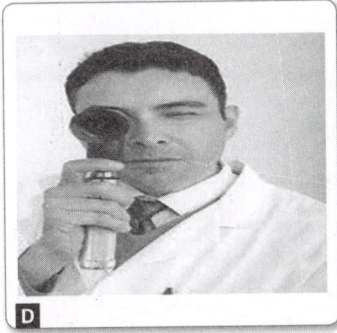 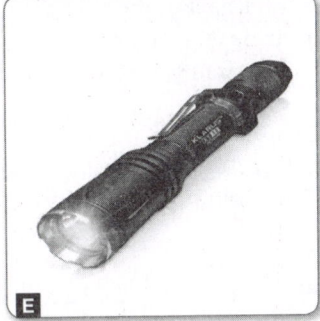 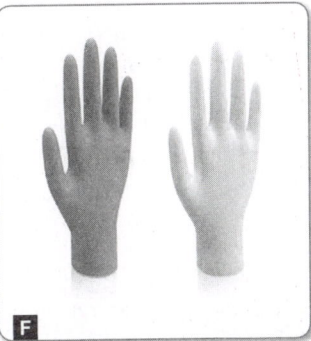

FIGS 1A TO F: A. Glucometer; **B.** Thermometer; **C.** Tuning fork; **D.** Ophthalmoscope; **E.** Torch; **F.** Disposable gloves

Sequence of Examination

- First of all examine the vital signs
- Auscultation may be done (Fig. 2)
- The examination should after that be followed by inspection, palpation, percussion, manipulation, recording of vital signs, elicitation of deep tendon reflexes, ENT examination and examination of painful site should be done at last.

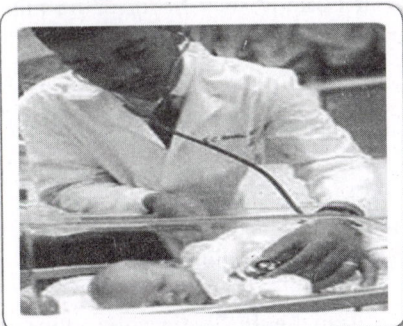

FIG. 2: Auscultation

MEASUREMENT OF VITAL SIGNS

Vital signs include temperature, pulse, respiration and blood pressure.

Articles Needed

A clean tray containing:
- Thermometer
- Digital and glass thermometers, disposable or single-use plastic thermometer strips and infrared thermometer
- A bottle containing antiseptic solution
- A bottle containing plain water
- A small bowl containing dry and wet cotton swabs .
- Kidney tray or paper bag
- TPR chart, pen and paper
- Wrist watch with seconds
- A stethoscope of pediatric size
- Alcohol swabs for cleaning the ear piece and chest piece
- Blood pressure cuff (appropriate size for the child)
- Doppler or electronic monitor or sphygmomanometer.

Temperature

Sites of checking temperature include oral, axillary, tympanic and rectal
- Never leave the child alone while taking temperature.
- Keep the thermometer in hand when it is in place for security and safety.
- Record the temperature.
- Report any elevated/subnormal temperature.
- Check the accuracy of any temperature if this does not correlate with the child's signs and symptoms.
- Wear gloves at the time of rectal temperature.

Steps of Checking Temperature

- Take thermometer out of box and hold at broad end
- Clean the shining tip with cotton spirit and wait till it dries
- Check the position of column of mercury
- If it is above the junction of the bulb with the stem then shake it gently by flicking at the wrist till the mercury in the column falls back into the chamber
- Remove/expose the baby's arm fully
- Place the silver bulb end of the thermometer under the baby's arm at the apex of the axilla, parallel to the lateral wall of the chest of the baby
- Gently hold the baby's arm against the body
- Keep the thermometer for 5 minutes
- Remove the thermometer and read the temperature
- Record the findings
- Inform the mother
- Clean the shining tip with cotton spirit and place it in the box

Temporal Scanning

- It is a newer method of temperature measurement that uses infrared scanning on the skin over the temporal artery combined with a mathematical computation to determine the child's arterial temperature.
- The arterial temperature is considered the most accurate reflection of body temperature.
- It measures the temperature on the exposed side of the head.
- Slide the sensor's tip externally in a horizontal line across the child's forehead, midway between the eyebrows and hairline and ending at the temporal artery.
- Hold it there until the device registers the temperature, which usually requires one second.
- Accuracy may be affected by excessive sweating.

Pulse

Sites

- Apical pulse
- Carotid pulse
- Brachial pulse
- Femoral pulse
- Popliteal pulse
- Posterior tibial pulse
- Dorsalis pedis pulse.

Procedure

- Take apical pulse rate of an infant.
- Place the stethoscope between the left nipple and sternum.
- Take heart rate for 1 minute.
- For older children, radial, temporal or carotid pulse may be taken.
- Try to take the pulse at the time of taking temperature.
- Record rate, rhythm (regular/irregular), strength of beat (full/bounding/weak/faint) and activity of child at the time of taking pulse (sleeping/crying)
- Report immediately if any abnormality is present.

Respiration (Fig. 3)

- Observe the chest movement for 1 minute
- Obtain respiration after checking temperature
- Note the observations and record
- Notice respiratory rate, depth, quality, sign of dyspnea, wheezing sound, etc.
- Report immediately if any abnormality is present.

Blood Pressure

- Site for checking blood pressure
  - Upper arm: 2 cm above antecubital fossa; auscultation area is brachial artery
  - Lower arm/forearm: 2 cm above wrist; auscultation area is radial artery
  - Thigh: 2 cm above the popliteal fossa; auscultation area is popliteal artery
  - Calf/ankle: 2 cm above ankle; auscultation area is posterior tibial dorsalis pedis artery

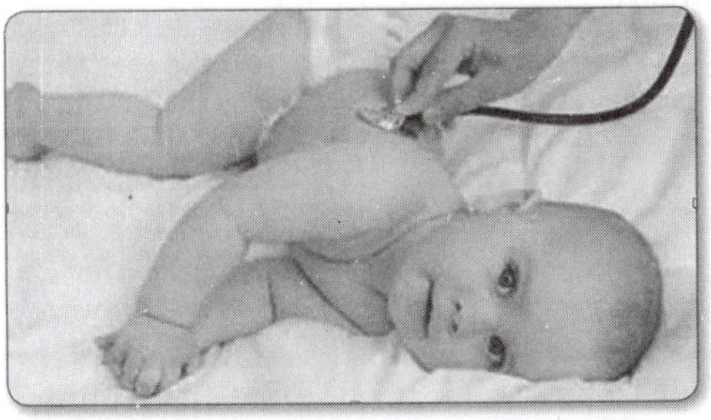

FIG. 3: Checking respiration (wheezing sign)

- The cuff should not be less than 1/2 and not more than 2/3 of the length of the upper arm or legs. Small variation of the cuff could provide a different measurement.
  - Too small cuff produces increased blood pressure.
  - Too wide cuff produces decreased blood pressure.
- If the child is excited at the person taking blood pressure, then systolic blood pressure may increase.
- BP varies with age, weight and height.
- Cuff should be according to the age of the child.

Examination of Skin (Figs 4A and B)

- Observe the skin color, pigmentation, jaundice, cyanosis, color of mucous membrane and hair disturbances
- Describe any variation in color with increased decreased pigmentation
- Record birth marks
- Observe unusual marks, any kind of wound, insect bites, etc.

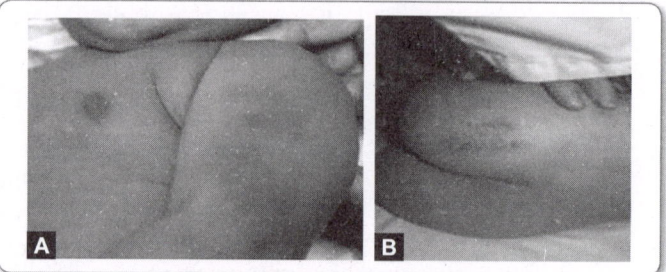

FIGS 4A AND B: Examination of skin

- Assess jaundice and color of skin
- The skin of new born infant will still be covered with vernix caseosa
- Note the presence of striae

Palpation

- Use tip of finger
- Feel tension of skin by pinching up a fold of skin
- Feel the skin texture, moisture and temperature tenderness.

Nails

Observe color, shape, irregularities in surface and cleanliness.

Hair

- Observe color and distribution according to age
- Be aware that tufts of hair over the spinal area may mark any abnormality
- Palpate the hair for texture and thickness
- Examine any patches where hair is missing
- Check scalp for any sign of lice infestation
- Inspect axilla and pubis

EXAMINATION OF HEAD AND NECK (FIGS 5A AND B)

- Observe the face and skin for asymmetry, deformity and abnormality
- Closely observe facial expression, blinking and crying
- Observe movement of head on the neck as the baby looks around, positions and moves
- Folds of skin should be carefully observed to ensure it is clear as free of perspiration rash or irritation.

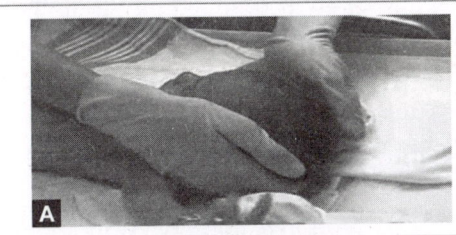 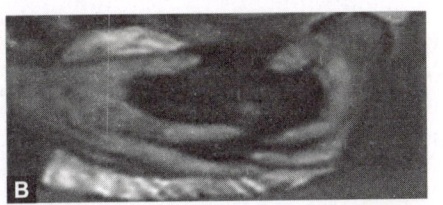

FIGS 5A AND B: Examination of head

- Pay particular attention to lachrymal duct
- Observe the distance between eyes the distribution of eyebrows
- Test the eyes for light perception.

Palpation

- If the child is old enough, have him squeeze his eye
- Check the quality.

Examination of Ears (Fig. 6)

- Examine external ear, the auricle, pinna and note the position of ear
- With free hand, pull the pinna back and slightly upward to straighten the canal, for examination
- Inspect the eardrum and test the mobility by means of a pneumatoscope
- Palpate behind the ear over the mastoid process.

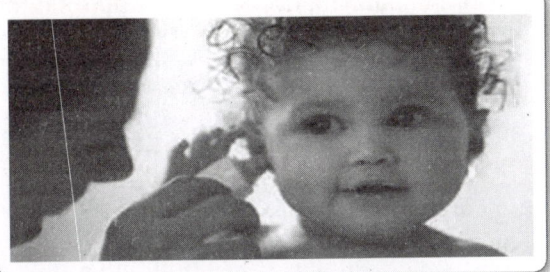

FIG. 6: Examination of ears

Examination of Nose

- Observe general deformity
- Examine nasal septum, mucous membrane and turbinate with a nasoscope and also examine any discharge obstruction
- Check the presence of any foreign bodies.

Examination of Mouth and Throat

- Observe the lips and note their color
- Count teeth, extra or missing, evidence of caries, staining tartar, malocclusion

- Check gums for swelling, bleeding and odor
- Check tongue movement, color, presence of taste buds, and frenulum as the gag reflex is elicited
- Note how the palate moves upward and uvula springs into view
- Inspect the heights of arch of palate.
- Note tonsils, position, surface, size, equality and color
- As the baby cries, note odor, hoarseness of voice, croup and wheezing:

TABLE 1: Eruption of teeth

Primary (Deciduous) Teeth		
Maxillary	**Eruption**	**Shedding**
• Central incisor	7 ½ months	7–8 years
• Lateral incisor	9 months	8–9 years
• Canine	18 months	11–12 years
• First molar	14 months	10–11 years
• Second molar	24 months	10–12 years
Mandibular		
• Central incisor	6 ½ months	6–7 years
• Lateral incisor	7 months	7–8 years
• Canine	16 months	9–11 years
• First molar	12 months	10--12 years
• Second molar	20 months	11–13 years
Permanent Teeth		
Maxillary	**Eruption**	
• Central incisor	7–8 years	
• Lateral incisor	8–9 years	
• Canine	11–12 years	
• First premolar	10–11 years	
• Second premolar	10–12 years	
• First molar	6–7 years	
• Second molar	12–13 years	
• Third molar	13–17 years	
Mandibular		
• Central incisor	6–7 years	
• Lateral incisor	7–8 years	
• Canine	9–10 years	
• First premolar	10–12 years	
• Second premolar	11–12 years	
• First molar	6–7 years	
• Second molar	11–13 years	
• Third molar	13–17 years	

EXAMINATION OF BREAST AND THORAX (FIG. 7)

- Check, if a small extra nipple is present
- Check, if the newborn's nipple appears a little darker than normal and breast tissue underneath may be from a small not with occasional leakage of milk
- Watch for any limp under the nipple
- Observe the entire thorax as the child breathes; note symmetry and equal expansion of both sides as the lungs inflate
- In thin children, the apical beat or the point of maximal impulse (PMI) can be easily seen
- Move the stethoscope in small jumps from the apical area medially towards the sternum. Go up to the left side of the sternum, listening to each interspace next to the sternum
- Move next to the patient's right second intercostal space again next to the sternum
- Descend down the right side of the sternum
- If there is any quest of heart murmur or added sounds, refer to the physician
- If the patient breaths in and out deeply, sinus arrhythmia will be obvious
- If a child holds his breath, the sinus arrhythmia will disappear. As you listen to the heart sound, you are also listening to the rhythm to confirm your finding
- In the infant, heart sounds are just a series of tapes, which occur so fast that it is impossible to make out which sounds is the first heart sound.

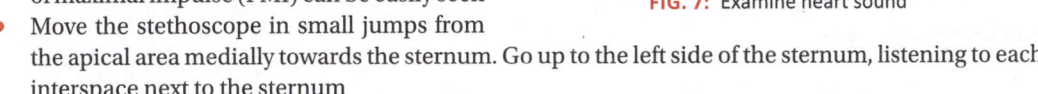

FIG. 7: Examine heart sound

EXAMINATION OF ABDOMEN

- Observe the abdomen for contour in standing and lying conditions. Inspect the respiration and movement of abdomen
- Check the early diagnosis of puberty
- Carefully inspect the umbilicus for cleanliness and presence of scar tissue.

TABLE 2: Different positions used for examining the children

0–3 months	Examination table
3 months to 1 year	Mother's lap
1–3 years	Standing or mother's lap
Greater than 3 years	Examination table

NEUROLOGICAL ASSESSMENT

Neurological assessment is based on neurological examination and four fundamental observations, which include assessment of reflex, muscle strength, cerebellar function, Glasgow coma scale and cranial nerves.

INDICATIONS

- Brain injury
- Intracranial tumors
- Neurologic conditions (e.g. meningitis and encephalitis)
- After cranial surgery.

COMPONENTS OF ASSESSMENT

- Level of consciousness (orientation and cognition)
- Pupillary signs (size, reactivity to light, quality of reaction)
- Motor tone and strength (hand grasp, pronator drift, leg movement and motor strength of extremities).

ARTICLES NEEDED

A clean tray containing the following:
- Measuring tape
- Reflex hammer
- Penlight
- Blunt tip needle
- Cotton swab
- Toys for children to play (crayons, paper, blocks, colorful pictures, books, ball and play dolls)
- Common scents
- Vision chart
- Flavors (salt, sugar and lemon)
- Tongue blade.

PRELIMINARY ASSESSMENT

- Assess the child's previous neurologic, general health, nutritional and developmental history.
- Assess the family understanding of current health status of the child.

PREPARATION

- Explain the procedure to the parents and the child and the purpose of neurological examination
- Collect medical history and previous neurological assessments to create baseline data
- Review the child's medical diagnosis, developmental and health history to determine whether any neurologic changes may be consistent with current health problems or medical history.

PROCEDURE

- Conduct neurological examination by assessing the higher mental functions such as the level of consciousness, intelligence, orientation to time, place, person, speech and observe the gait
- Measure the head circumference and inspect the child's cranial shape for symmetry and palpate fontanels to assess whether they are open, note if they are sunken or bulging
- Observe the child at rest, noting his/her behavior and mood. Respond to surroundings and movements.

- Inspect the child's skin, noting neurocutaneous findings, such as sacral dimples, spine curvature, hemangiomas, etc.

CRANIAL NERVES ASSESSMENT

- **Perception of smell-I:** Ask the child to identify some common odorous material (e.g. orange and chocolate with his/her eyes closed).
- **Perception of vision-II:** >3 years: The vision can be screened by the use of Snellen chart.
  - To check blinking response of children to bright light, turn the head towards diffuse light or follow red moving ball or ring.
  - The visual acuity in a term newborn baby is around 6/45, and it gradually matures to an adult level of 6/6 by the age of 6–7 years.
  - To test the field of vision for >3 years, an object suspended from a thread is gradually brought from the periphery towards the eye and the child is asked to indicate when the object is visualized.
  - **Color vision:** >3 years: By showing different color objects.
  - Infant's Doll's eye movement phenomenon is used to test the ocular movements.
- **Hearing-VIII:** Enquire any hearing defect, tinnitus, vertigo, and dizziness. Ask for response of the child to noise of jet plane, banging of door, music and calling of his name, etc. Use Weber's test or Rinne's test.
- **Taste-VII:** Assess taste by asking to discern certain common tastes (sugar and salt)
- **Movements of Eyeballs:** III, IV, VI: Look for squint, movements of eyeballs, diplopia and nystagmus. The child is asked to look at the examiner's fingers which are moved slowly horizontally in either direction and vertically up and down.
- Infant's Doll's eye movement phenomenon is used to test the ocular movements.
- **Face-VII:** Note symmetry of facial expressions.
- **Muscles of Mastication-V:** Infant: Note strength of infant's sucking refer of pacifier, examiner's thumb or bottle. Assess the strength of bite of the child and his/her ability to discern light touch on the face.
- **Tongue—Swallowing and Gag Reflex-IX, X:** Ask the child to identify different tastes on the back of the tongue and tell the child to swallow. A tongue blade may be used to elicit the gag reflex.
- XII: Ask the child to stick out his/her tongue and instruct him/her to speak.

CEREBELLAR FUNCTION

- Balance, gait and leg coordination, ataxia, posture, tremors
- Finger to nose (fingers to thumb): 3–4 years
- Finger to examiner's finger: 4–6 years
- Rapid alternations of hands (prone, supine): School age
- Tandem walk: 4–6 years
- Walk on toes, heels: School age
- Stand on one foot: 3–6 years
- Ask the child to stand with feet together, arms at sides and eyes closed, like a soldier to elicit Romberg's sign.

MOTOR SYSTEM

- Assess the following for upper and lower limbs: Size, tone, power of the muscle and reflexes. The power of muscle strength is checked by assessing the grip strength, individual muscle strength and assessment findings are generally graded from 0 to 5
    - 0: No movements
    - 1: Trace muscle contraction
    - 2: Active movement
    - 3: Active movement against gravity
    - 4: Active movement against gravity resistance
    - 5: Normal power of movement
- Ask the child to squeeze your fingers
- Ask the child to make muscles by bending arms at elbows with palms facing body and resist your attempt to straighten arm to assess biceps strength
- **Triceps:** Ask the child to extend arms and resist your attempt to flex or bend arm
- **Quadriceps:** While the child is seated with legs dangling bed or table, asks the child to extend each leg straight and resist your attempt to bend legs
- **Gastrocnemius muscle:** Ask the child to press the sole of foot against your hand
- **Tibial–radialis strength:** Ask the child to bend toes up toward his/her face while you place your hand on top of foot
- **To detect spasticity:** Passively move the child's extremities, noting tone and ease of movement
- Ask the child to draw a picture and build a tower of blocks
- Ask the child to pick up a small object, observing finger and hand movements bilaterally.

Reflex Assessment

- **Biceps:** Flex the child's fore arm, place your thumb over the child's antecubital space and tap with reflex hammer. **Response:** Slight flexion at the arm when the tendon is tapped.
- **Triceps:** Abduct the child's arm and support forearm with your hand or hold child's wrist over his/her chest to flex arm at the elbow. Tap directly above the elbow. Response: partial extension
- **Brachioradialis tendon:** Place the child's arm and hand in relaxed position with arm flexed and palm down. Tap the radius about 1 inch above the wrist. Response: Flexion of forearm and upward turn of the palm.
- **Patellar:** Use reflex hammer to tap the front outer aspect of the child's knee, midline, just below patella when the child is sitting on the edge of the table or bed with the leg dangling. Response: Slight extension.
- **Achilles tendon:** Assist the child to a seated position on the edge of a table or bed. The child's legs should dangle freely over the edge. Support child's foot at the 90-degree angle and use reflex hammer to tap the back of child's heel. If the child is in supine position, flex one leg at knee and hip supporting the lower position of that leg on the opposite side. Lightly support foot in your hand in dorsiflexion and tap Achilles tendon. Response: Plantar flexion.
- **Babinski sign:** Strike the outer sole of the child's foot from heel to toes with the handle of reflex hammer and note movement of toes. Response: In children older than 2 years of age, the toes should flex downward.

Upward movement of the big toe with other toes fanning outward.

- **Kernig's sign:** With child lying supine, lift child's leg with flexion at knee and hip. Note any pain or resistance
- **Brudzinski's sign:** An involuntary flexion of the hip and knees when neck is passively flexed
- **Anal reflex:** Gently stroke the perianal skin. Contracture of anal sphincter
- **Abdominal reflex:** With child lying supine, stroke abdominal skin in all four quadrants by moving handle of reflex hammer from the side towards the midline
- **Cremasteric reflex:** Gently stroke the inner aspect of a male child's thigh, the testis of the side of the stroked thigh should retract into inguinal canal.

TABLE 3: Pediatric glasgow coma scale (modified)

Activity	Best response	Score
Eye opening	• Spontaneous	4
	• To voice	3
	• To pain	2
	• None	1
Verbal response (V)	• Smiles, oriented to sounds, follows objects, interacts	5
	• Cries but consolable, inappropriate interactions	4
	• Inconsistently inconsolable, moaning	3
	• Inconsolable, agitated	2
	• None	1
Motor response (M)	• Moves spontaneously or purposefully	6
	• Withdraws from touch	5
	• Withdraws to pain	4
	• Decorticates posture (an abnormal posture that can include rigidity, clenched fists, legs held straight out, and arms bent inward toward the body with the wrists and fingers bend and held on the chest)	3
	• Decerebrate (an abnormal posture that can include rigidity, arms and legs held straight out, toes pointed downward, head and neck arched backward)	2
	• None	1

Pediatric brain injuries are classified by severity using the same scoring levels as adults.

TABLE 4: Score chart for pediatric brain injuries

3–8	Most severe injury
9–12	Moderate injury
13–15	Mild injury

DEVELOPMENTAL ASSESSMENT

INTRODUCTION

Developmental assessment includes early identification of problems through screening and surveillance, and more definitive assessment including both standardized and nonstandardized measures, as well as integration of information from the developmental, social, and family history and the medical history and examination.

GOALS OF DEVELOPMENTAL ASSESSMENT

- The goal of developmental assessment is not only to generate a diagnosis, but it is equally important to analyze the pattern of strengths and weaknesses in the child, family and available developmental, educational, and social support systems, in order to direct treatment.
- The maturation of the central nervous system (CNS) is characterized by coordination of motor activity, and as infants grow they respond to their environment in a purposeful manner with the help of special senses (acoustic and auditory inputs), integrity of labyrinthine, vestibular and musculoskeletal systems.
- Children achieve neuromotor milestones of development at predictable ages within a narrow range of a few weeks or months.
- Development is dependent upon the interaction between innate genetic potential and environmental factors such as emotional security, love and attention, stimulating home environment, optimal nutrition and ethnic and cultural factors.
- Neuromotor retardation may occur due to gestational immaturity, perinatal hypoxia, birth trauma, metabolic disorders (inborn errors of metabolism), hypoglycemia, kernicterus, intrauterine infections, postnatal CNS infections, hypothyroidism and developmental and chromosomal disorders.

PRINCIPLES OF DEVELOPMENT

- Development it is the most distinctive attribute of childhood and is a continuous process from conception to maturity
- It is intimately related to the maturation of the CNS
- The sequence of development is identical in all children, but the rate of development varies from child to child
- The child with an odd-looking face does not necessarily have associated mental subnormality
- The attributes such as creativity, future potentiality, IQ and mental superiority cannot be predicted in an individual child by developmental assessment
- The generalized mass activity of early infancy is replaced by specific and subtle individual responses
- It is a common observation that when an infant is shown a bright object, it shows wild excitement by moving trunk, arms, legs and babbling while an older child merely smiles and reaches for the object
- The development proceeds in a cephalocaudal direction. The infant initially develops head control followed by ability to roll over, grasp, sitting, crawling, standing, walking, etc
- Certain primitive reflexes such as grasp reflex and walking reflex must be lost before corresponding voluntary movements are required.

PURPOSE

The main purpose of developmental assessment depends on the age of the child:
- Tests may detect neurological problems such as cerebral palsy in the neonate
- Tests may reassure parents or detect problems in early infancy
- Testing in late childhood can help detect academic and social problems early enough to minimize possible negative consequences (although parental concern may be just as good a predictor for some problems)

- No developmental screening tool can allow for the dynamic nature of child development. A child's performance on one particular day is influenced by many factors. Development is not a linear process, it is characterized by spurts, plateau and sometimes regressions
- Gradually, screening has how been replaced by the concept of developmental surveillance. This is a much broader concept. It involves parents, allows for context and should be a flexible, continuous process.

DIFFERENT DOMAINS OF DEVELOPMENT

- Gross motor development
- Fine motor development
- Social/cognitive/intellectual development
- Speech and language development
- Vision and hearing development.

GROSS MOTOR DEVELOPMENT

- The acquisition of gross motor skill precedes the development of fine motor skills
- Both processes occur in a cephalocaudal fashion
- Head control preceding arm and hand control
- Followed by leg and foot control.

SUSPENSION POSITION

The examiner suspends the infant in a prone position by supporting the abdomen of the baby on his palm. The extension of neck and flexion of the extremities is observed.
- Newborn: Head hangs completely and back is rounded
- Four weeks: Head momentarily lifted up, elbow flexed
- Six weeks: Head held momentarily in the same plane as the rest of the body
- Eight weeks: Head maintained in the same plane as the rest of the body and momentarily lifted beyond this
- Twelve weeks: Head maintained well beyond the plane of the rest of the body.

PRONE POSITION

The infant is placed in a prone position on a clean place, when we observed the following:
- Newborn: Head is kept to one side, pelvis is raised and knees are drawn up under the abdomen
- 4–6 weeks: Hips and knees are partially extended, can lift chin off the couch momentarily
- Eight weeks: Head is maintained in midline with chin lifted off the couch
- Sixteen weeks: Chest is maintained off the couch and arms are stretched out in full extension
- Twenty weeks: The body is supported on forearms
- Twenty-four weeks: Weight is supported on hands, and baby rolls prone to supine.

SUPINE POSTURE AND SITTING

The infant is placed supine on the couch and pulled to sitting position by lifting at the forearms (traction response).
- Newborn: Complete head lag

- Four weeks: Head maintained in plane of the body momentarily when the baby is held in a sitting position; back is rounded. Chin may be lifted up momentarily
- Twelve weeks: Head held up when supported in a position but it tends to bob (bend) forwards
- Sixteen weeks: When pulled up, there is slight head lag during the beginning and then head is flexed beyond the plane of the body. When held in sitting position and the baby is swayed (swung), the head wobbles
- Twenty weeks: No head lag; head is stable without wobbling (shaking) and back is straight
- Twenty-four weeks: When about to be pulled up, lifts head off the couch in anticipation. Can sit with a support in a pram (baby carriage) or high chair
- Twenty-eight weeks: Can sit on the floor with hands forward for support
- Thirty-two weeks: Can sit momentarily on the floor without support
- Thirty-six weeks: Sits steadily without support and can lean forward and recover his balance
- Forty weeks: Can sit up from supine position
- Forty-eight weeks: Can turn sideways and twist around to pick up an object.

VENTRAL SUSPENSION, STANDING AND WALKING

- Newborn: Walking reflex for 2–3 weeks
- Eight weeks: Can hold head up more than momentarily
- Twenty-four weeks: Puts almost all weight of the body on the legs
- Twenty-eight weeks: Bounces with pleasure
- Thirty-six weeks: Pulls self to stand, can stand with support
- Forty-four weeks: Lifts one foot while standing
- One year: Walks two hands held or on holding the furniture
- Fifteen months: Walks a few steps independently. Creeps upstairs and can kneel without support
- Eighteen months: Can get up and down the stairs without help, pull a wheeled toy
- Two years: Walks up and down the stairs with two feet on each step, walks backwards on imitation, picks up objects from floor without falling, runs and can kick a ball
- Two and half years: Can walk tiptoed, jumps on both feet
- Three years: Goes upstairs with one foot on each step, jumps off the bottom step
- Four years: Comes downstairs with one foot on each step; can skip on one foot
- Five years: Skips on both feet.

FINE MOTOR DEVELOPMENT

Fine motor skill is the coordination of small muscles, in movements—usually involving the synchronization of hands and fingers—with the eyes

- Newborn has very little control. Objects will be involuntarily grasped and dropped without notice.
- Four months: Bidextrous reach
- Six months: Undexterous reach; transfer object
- Nine months: Immature pincer grasp; probes with forefinger
- Twelve months: Pincer grasp mature
- Fifteen months: Imitates scribbling; tower of 2 blocks
- Eighteen months: Scribbles; tower of 3 blocks
- Two years: Tower of 6 blocks; vertical and circular stroke

- Three years: Tower of 9 blocks; copies circle
- Four years: Copies cross; bridge with blocks
- Five years: Copies triangle.

SOCIAL/COGNITIVE/INTELLECTUAL DEVELOPMENT

- Observe exploration and free play, use of real size and small toys on self and others and initiation and response to social games (e.g. peek-a-boo, pat-a-cake)
- Note initiating interactions and responding to parent/examiner/other children and use of eye contact and gestures.
- Two months: Social smile
- Three months: Recognizes mother; anticipates feeds
- Six months: Recognizes strange/stranger anxiety
- Nine months: Waves 'bye-bye'
- Twelve months: Comes when called; plays simple ball game
- Eighteen months: Jargon
- Eighteen months: Copies parents in task
- Two years: Asks for food, drink, toilet; pulls people to show toys
- Three years: Shares toys; knows full name and gender
- Four years: Plays cooperatively in a group; goes to toilet alone
- Five years: Helps in household tasks; dresses and undresses.

SPEECH AND LANGUAGE DEVELOPMENT

- Observes vocalization and gestures to attract other's attention, to indicate needs. Responses to others' vocalization and shares emotions
- Notes speech quality, use of language to express need, comment, describe, shares interest and initiates and responds to conversation
- One month: Alert to sound
- Three months: Coo
- Four months: Laughs loud
- Six months: Monosyllables
- Nine months: Learns bisyllables
- Twelve months: 1–2 words with meaning
- Eighteen months: 8–10 words vocabulary
- Two years: 2–3 words sentence, use pronouns "I", "me", and "you"
- Three years: Asks questions; knows full name and gender
- Four years: Says song or poem; tells stories
- Five years: Asks meaning of words.

VISION AND HEARING DEVELOPMENT

Hearing

Prenatal Stimulation

- The human fetus possesses rudimentary hearing from 20 weeks of gestation. This hearing will develop and mature during the remainder of gestation. The fetus is able to hear sounds outside the mother's body, although he or she is able to hear low-frequency sounds much better than high-frequency sounds.

The First Two Important Years

- The first two years is the time during which hearing develops in children. It is important for parents to be able to recognize signs of a hearing problem as early as possible and seek medical attention if there are any concerns.

Four Months

- Move or react when someone speaks or in response to any noise
- Startle when there is a very loud noise.

Seven Months

- Turn his/her head towards a voice or a noise (when a parent calls even without being seen)
- Stirs or moves in response to a noise or voice
- Startles when there is a large sound.

Nine Months

Turns his/her head to find out from where a sound is coming:
- Turn around if a parent is calling from behind
- Stir or move in response to voice or sound
- Startle when there is a very loud noise.

Twelve Months

- Turn his/her head in all directions and show an interest in a person's voice or a particular sound
- Repeat sounds that parents make
- Startle in response to a loud noise.

Vision

At Birth

- **The irises:** The iris lacks pigment and may have a grey or bluish appearance; natural color develops as pigment forms
- The eyes' pupils are not able to dilate fully yet
- The curvature of the lens: is nearly spherical not oval
- The retina (especially the macula) is not fully developed
- The sight: The newborn has poor fixation ability, a very limited ability to discriminate color, limited visual fields.

One Month

- The infant can follow a slowly moving black and white target intermittently to midline
- May also intermittently follow faces (usually with the eyes and head both moving together)
- She/he will blink at a light flash
- There is a preference for black and white designs.

Two Months

- Brief fixation occurs sporadically, ocular movements are still uncoordinated
- The infant follows vertical movements better than horizontal
- Begins to be aware of colors (primarily red and yellow)
- There is probably still a preference for black and white designs.

Three Months

- Ocular movements are coordinated most of the time; attraction is to both black and white and colored (yellow and red) targets
- The infant is capable of glancing at smaller targets and is interested in faces; visual attention and visual searching begins
- The infant begins to associate visual stimuli and an event (e.g. the bottle and feeding).

Four Months

- "Hand regard" occurs; there is marked interest in the infant's own hands
- He/she is beginning to shift gaze and reacts (usually smiles) to familiar faces
- He/she is able to follow a visual target past midline and can track horizontally, vertically and in a circle.

Five Months

- Eye–hand coordination (reach) is usually achieved by now
- The infant is able to look at an object in his/her own hands
- The infant is visually aware of the environment ("explores" visually) and can easily shift gaze from near to far.

Six Months

- Eye movements are coordinated and smooth; vision can be used efficiently at both a near point and distance
- The child recognizes and differentiates faces and can reach for and grasp a visual target
- Hand movements are monitored visually; has visually directed reach
- May be interested in watching falling objects and usually fixates on where the object disappears.

Between 6 and 9 Months

- Acuity improves rapidly (to near normal)
- "Explores" visually (examines objects in hands visually and watches what is going on around him/her)
- Can transfer objects from hand to hand and may be interested in geometric patterns.

Between 9 Months and a Year

The child can visually spot a small (2–3 mm) object nearby

- Watches faces and tries to imitate expressions
- Searches for hidden objects
- Is visually alert to new people, objects, and surroundings
- Can differentiate between known and unfamiliar people.

One Year

- Mild farsightedness
- Ability to focus, accommodate (shift between far and near vision tasks)
- He/she can discriminate between simple geometric forms (circle, triangle, square), scribbles with a crayon and is visually interested in pictures.

Two Years

- Myelinization of the optic nerve is completed
- All optical skills are smooth and well-coordinated
- The child can imitate movements, can match same objects by single properties (color and shape), and can point to specific pictures in a book.

Three Years

- Retinal tissue is mature
- The child can complete a simple form board correctly (based on visual memory)
- Can do simple puzzles, can draw a crude circle, and can put 1 inch things into holes.

DEVELOPMENTAL QUOTIENT (DQ) AND INTELLIGENT QUOTIENT

The child may be assigned a DQ after clinical assessment of development in children with development delay.

$$DQ = \frac{\text{Developmental age}}{\text{Chronological age}} \times 100$$

DQ Interpretation

- Maximum score = 100
- ≥ 85: Normal
- 71–84: Mild-to-moderate delay
- ≤ 70: Severe delay

Intelligence is related to developments in various do mains, but it is not the same as development. Intelligence does not just include performing the given task, but it also includes the ability to understand and reason out the task.

$$IQ = \frac{\text{Mental age}}{\text{Chronological age}} \times 100$$

TABLE 5: Interpretation of intelligence quotient

IQ Levels		Interpretation of intelligence
Below 20	—	Profound mental retardation (MR)
20–25	—	Severe MR
35–50	—	Moderate MR
50–70	—	Mild MR
91–110	—	Slow learner
111–120	—	Average
121–140	—	Superior
Above 140	—	Gifted

EXAMINATION: OBSERVATIONS AND INTERACTIVE ASSESSMENT

- It should take place in a room appropriate for a child
- It could be with one or both parents, but they should not prompt and help the child
- Chair and table: Child's behavior and interaction with parents during history taking should be observed prior to physical examination
- Normal functioning of motor, vision and hearing should be assessed.

Articles Required

- A red ring
- A small bell
- Pellet made of card board, wool or paper (8 mm size)
- 10 cubes of 1 inch each (colorful)
- A pen and paper
- A picture book of common objects
- Card with circle, cross, square, triangle drawn on them
- Rattle
- Bunch of keys
- Cup with handle
- Beads
- Paper and crayons
- Red ball.

Time of Assessment

- Developmental surveillance
- Child visit

Developmental Screening Charts

- Sophisticated developmental testing instruments are time consuming and require the services of a trained developmental psychologist.
- They are useful for detection of borderline abnormalities as well as for research purposes.
- There is a need to develop reliable simple developmental charts which can be used by a medical health worker or clinician of the related field.
- **Examples**
  - Denver developmental screening test
  - Bayley developmental screening chart
  - Trivandrum development screening chart
  - Seguin form board
  - Vineland social maturity scale

Denver Developmental Screening Test

- Denver development screening test (DDST) is a widely used assessment for examining the developmental progress of children from birth until the age of 6, developed in 1967.
- Concerns were raised about specific items in the test and, coupled with changing normal values, it was decided that a major revision of the test was necessary in 1992.

Test design

- The test consists of up to 125 items, divided into four parts (ages covered by the tests range from birth to 6 years):
    - Gross motor functions: Motor control, sitting, walking, jumping and other movements.
    - Fine motor function: Eye/hand coordination and manipulation of small objects, e.g. grasping and drawing.
    - Language: Production of sounds, ability to recognize, understand, and use of language, e.g. ability to combine words.
    - Social/personal: Aspects of socialization inside and outside the home, e.g. smiling.

Application

- No special training is required
- The test takes approximately 20 minutes to administer and interpret
- There may be some variation in time taken, depending on both the age and cooperation of the child
- Interviews can be performed by almost anyone who works with children and medical professionals
- The items are recorded through direct observations of the child plus, for some points, the mother reports whether the child is capable of performing a given task
- Younger infants can sit on their mother's lap
- The test should be given slowly.

Interpretation of the test

- The data is presented as age norms, similar to a growth curve
- Draw a vertical line at the child's chronological age on the charts; if the infant is premature, subtract the months premature from chronological age
- The more items a child fails to perform (passed by 90% of his/her peers), the more likely the child manifests a significant developmental deviation that warrants further evaluation.

Bayley Developmental Screening Chart

- Bayley development screening chart (BDSC) was first published by Nancy Bayley in *The Bayley Scales of Infant Development* (1969) and in the second edition in 1993
- The scale has been used extensively worldwide to assess the development of infants
- The test is given on an individual basis and takes 45–60 minutes to complete. It is administered by examiners who are experienced clinicians specifically trained in BSID test procedures. The examiner presents a series of test materials to the child and observes the child's responses and behaviors
- The test contains items designed to identify young children at risk for developmental delay
- The Bayley Scales of Infant Development (BSID) measures the mental and motor development and tests the behavior of infants from 1 to 42 months of age
- The BSID is used to describe the current developmental functioning of infants and to assist in diagnosis and treatment planning for infants with developmental delays or disabilities
- The test is intended to measure a child's level of development in three domains: cognitive, motor and behavioral.

BSID evaluates individuals along three scales:

- Mental scale: This part of the evaluation, which yields a score called the mental development index, evaluates several types of abilities: sensory/perceptual acuities, discriminations and response; acquisition of object constancy; memory learning and problem solving; vocalization and beginning of verbal communication; basis of abstract thinking; habituation; mental mapping; complex language; and mathematical concept formation

- Motor scale: This part of the BSID assesses the degree of body control, large muscle coordination, finer manipulative skills of the hands and fingers, dynamic movement, postural imitation and the ability to recognize objects by sense of touch (stereo gnosis)
- Behavior rating scale: This scale provides information that can be used to supplement information gained from the mental and motor scales. This 30-item scale rates the child's relevant behaviors and measures attention/arousal, orientation/engagement, emotional regulation, and motor quality
- The BSID are known to have high reliability and validity. The mental and motor scales have high correlation coefficients (0.83 and 0.77, respectively) for test–retest reliability.

Trivandrum Developmental Screening Chart

- Trivandrum development screening chart (TDSC) is suitable for developmental screening of children below 2 years by a paramedical health worker
- The range of each test item has been taken from the norms obtained on the Bayley scales of infant development
- It is based on 17 simple test items carefully chosen from among 67 motor items of Bayley scales of infant development (Baroda norms)
- The left-hand side of each horizontal dark line represents age at which 3% of children passed the item and the right edge represents the age at which 97% of the children passed the item in studies conducted at Trivandrum
- A plastic ruler or pencil is kept vertically at the level of chronological age of the child being tested If the child fails to pass any item that lies to the left side of the age marker, the child is considered to have developmental delay
- It is simple to use and takes 5 to 7 minutes to administer. It is best suited to use in infants around one year of age because most of the test items are concentrated around that age period.

Seguin Form Board

- The Seguin Form Board (SFB) is based on the single factor theory of intelligence which measures speed and accuracy
- It is useful in evaluating a child's eye–hand coordination, shape concept, visual perception and cognitive ability. The test is primarily used to assess visual–motor skills
- It includes Gesell figures wherein the child is asked to copy 10 geometrical figures to evaluate visual–motor ability. Test materials consist of 10 differently shaped wooden blocks and a large form board with recessed corresponding shapes.

Vineland Social Maturity Scale

- The Vineland Social Maturity Scale (VSMS) measures social competence, self-help skills and adaptive behavior from infancy to adulthood. It is used in planning for therapy and/or individualized instruction for persons with mental retardation or emotional disorders
- The VSMS, published by Edgar Doll in 1935, measures social maturity or social competence in individuals from birth to adulthood
- The Vineland scale, which can be used from birth up to the age of 30, consists of a 117-item interview with a parent or other primary caregiver. (There is also a classroom version for ages 3–12 years that can be completed by a teacher)

- Doll classified eight categories of items on the VSMS (Doll, 1935): Self-help general, self-help dressing, self-help eating, communication, self-direction, socialization, locomotion and occupation
- Although there is some difference of opinion as to whether Doll's categorization is the best, the perception of adaptive behavior as multidimensional has survive from one generation to the next
- The test is untimed and takes 20–30 minutes. Raw scores are converted to an age equivalent score (expressed as social age) and a social quotient
- Personal and social skills are evaluated in the following areas:
  - Daily living skills (general self-help, eating and dressing)
  - Communication (listening, speaking, writing)
  - Motor skills (fine and gross, including locomotion)
  - Socialization (interpersonal relationships, play and leisure and coping skills)
  - Occupational skills
  - Self-direction. (An optional maladaptive behavior scale is also available).

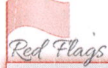

Red Flags

Birth to three months:
- Rolling prior to 3 months
- Evaluate for hypertonia
- Persistent fisting at 3 months
- Evaluate for neuromotor dysfunction
- Failure to alert to environmental stimuli
- Evaluate for sensory impairment

4–6 months
- Poor head control
- Evaluate for hypotonia
- Failure to reach for objects by 5 months
- Evaluate for motor, visual or cognitive deficits
- Absent smile
- Evaluate visual loss
- Evaluate attachment problems
- Evaluate maternal depression
- Consider child abuse or child neglect in severe cases

6–12 months
- Persistence of primitive reflexes after 6 months
- Evaluate for neuromuscular disorder
- Absent babbling by 6 months
- Evaluate for hearing deficit
- Absent stranger anxiety by 7 months
- May be related to multiple care providers
- Inability to localise sound by 10 months
- Evaluate for unilateral hearing loss
- Persistent mouthing of objects at 12 months
- May indicate lack of intellectual curiosity

12–24 months
Lack of consonant production by 15 months

Contd...

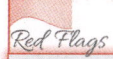
Red Flags

Evaluate mild hearing loss
Lack of imitation by 16 months
Evaluate hearing deficit
Evaluate cognitive or socialization deficit
Hand dominance prior to 18 months
May indicate contralateral weakness with hemiparesis
Inability to walk up and downstairs at 24 months
May lack opportunity rather than motor deficit
Advanced noncommunicative speech (e.g., echolalia)
Simple commands not understood suggests abnormality
Evaluate autism
Evaluate pervasive developmental disorder
Delayed language development
Requires hearing loss evaluation in all children

TABLE 6: Developmental milestones

Age	Motor	Speech	Vision and hearing	Social
1–1.5 months	When held upright, holds head erect and steady	Coos and babbles at parents and people they know	Focuses on parents	• Loves looking at new faces • Starts to smile at parents • Startled by sudden noises
1.6–2 months	When prone, lifts self by arms; rolls from side to back	Vocalizes; coos (makes vowel-like noises) or babbles	Focuses on objects as well as adults	• Loves looking at new faces • Smiles at parent • Starting to smile
2.1–4.5 months	• Rolls from tummy to side • Rests on elbows • Lifts head 90° • Sits propped up with hands, head steady for short time	• Changes sounds while verbalizing, 'eee-ahhh' • Verbalizes to engage someone in interaction • Blows bubbles, plays with tongue • Deep belly laughs	• Hand regard: following the hand with the eyes • Color vision adult-like	• Serves to practice emerging visual skills • Also observed in blind children
3 months	• Prone: head held up for prolonged periods • No grasp reflex	Makes vowel noises	• Follows dangling toy from side to side • Turns head round to sound • Follows adults' gaze • Sensitivity to binocular cues emerges	• Squeals with delight appropriately • Discriminates smile; Smiles often • Laughs at simple things • Reaches out for objects
5 months	• Holds head steady • Goes for objects and gets them • Objects taken to mouth	Enjoys vocal play		• Notices colors • Adjusts hand shape to shape of toy before picking up

Contd...

Age	Motor	Speech	Vision and hearing	Social
6 months	• Transfers objects from one hand to the other. Pulls self-up to sit and sits erect with supports • Rolls over prone to supine • Palmar grasp of cube hand-to-hand eye coordination	Double syllable sounds such as 'mumum' and 'dada'; babbles (consonant-vowel combinations)	• Localises sound 45 cm lateral to either ear • Visual acuity adult like (20/20) • Sensitivity to pictorial depth cues (those used by artists to indicate depth) emerges	May show stranger anxiety
9–10 months	• Wiggles and crawls • Sits unsupported • Picks up objects with pincer grasp	Babbles tunefully	Looks for toys dropped	Apprehensive about strangers
1 year	• Stands holding furniture • Stands alone for a second or two, then collapses with a bump	Babbles 2 or 3 words repeatedly	Drops toys and watches where they go	• Cooperates with dressing, waves goodbye, understands simple commands
18 months	• Can walk alone • Picks up toy without falling over. • Gets up/downstairs holding onto rail • Begins to jump with both feet • Can build tower of 3 or 4 cubes and throw a tower a ball	'Jargon'. Many intelligible words	Is able to recognize favorite songs, and will try to join in	• Demands constant mothering • Drinks from a cup with both hands • Feeds self with a spoon • Most children with autism are diagnosed at this age
2 years	• Able to run • Walks up and down stairs 2 feet per step. • Builds tower of 6 cubes	Joins 2–3 words in sentences		Parallel play. Day by day
3 years	• Goes up stairs 1-foot per step and downstairs 2 feet per step • Copies circle, imitates hand motions and draws man on request • Builds tower of 9 cubes	• **Constantly asks** questions • Speaks in sentences		• Cooperative play • Undresses with assistance • Imaginary companions
4 years	• Goes downstairs one foot per step, skips on one foot • Imitates gate with cubes, copies a cross	• **Questioning at its peak** • **Many** infantile substitutions **in speech**		• **Dresses and undresses with assistance** • **Attends to own** toilet **needs**

Contd…

Age	Motor	Speech	Vision and hearing	Social
5 years	• Skips on both feet and hops. Draws a man and copies a hexagonal-based pyramid using graphing paper • Gives age	• Fluent speech with few infantile substitutions in speech		Dresses and undresses alone

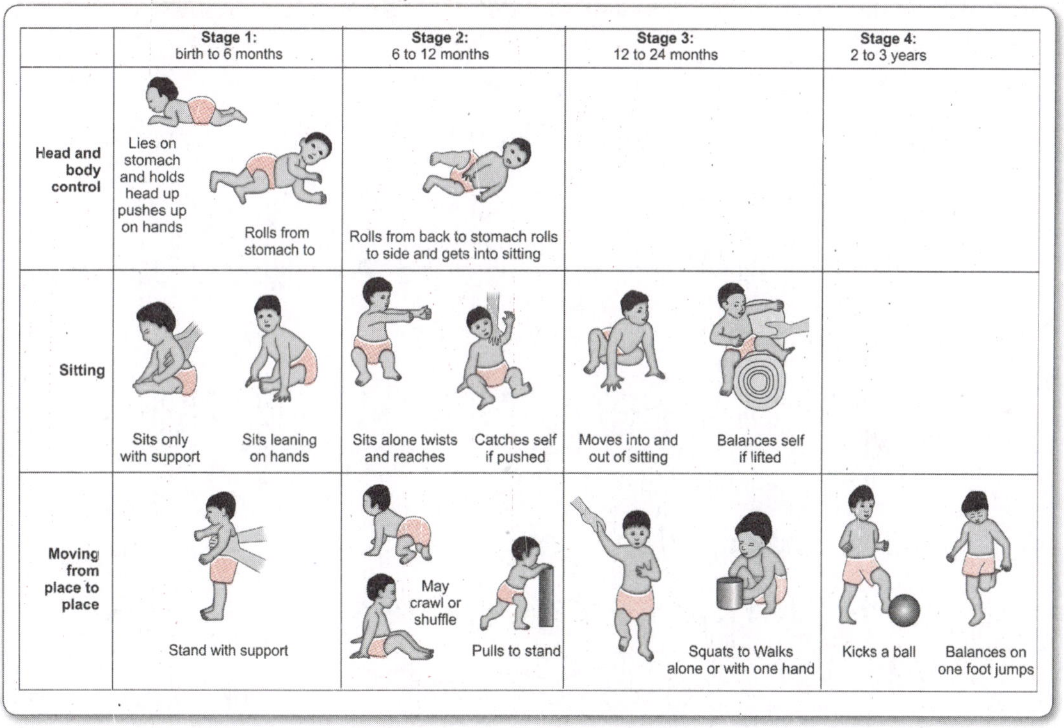

	Stage 1: birth to 6 months	Stage 2: 6 to 12 months	Stage 3: 12 to 24 months	Stage 4: 2 to 3 years
Head and body control	Lies on stomach and holds head up pushes up on hands Rolls from stomach to	Rolls from back to stomach rolls to side and gets into sitting		
Sitting	Sits only with support Sits leaning on hands	Sits alone twists and reaches Catches self if pushed	Moves into and out of sitting Balances self if lifted	
Moving from place to place	Stand with support	May crawl or shuffle Pulls to stand	Squats to Walks alone or with one hand	Kicks a ball Balances on one foot jumps

FIG. 8: Developmental milestones

5

Nutritional Assessment of Children

- ⮞ Nutritional Assessment
- ⮞ Breastfeeding
- ⮞ Formula Preparation and Artificial Feeding
- ⮞ Artificial Feeding
- ⮞ Katori and Spoon Feeding/Paladai Feeding
- ⮞ Complementary Feeding
- ⮞ Recommended Daily Dietary Allowances
- ⮞ Malnutrition Assessment

LEARNING OBJECTIVES

By the end of this chapter, the reader will be able to perform the following activities:
- Identify the different methods for assessing the nutritional status
- Assess the basic anthropometric techniques, applications and reference standards

NUTRITIONAL ASSESSMENT

PURPOSE

- To assess malnutrition
- To assess over- and undernutrition
- To prevent malnutrition
- To detect diseases and early treatment.

METHODS

There are two types of methods such as direct and indirect methods.

Direct Method

These are summarized as ABCD:
- **A**nthropometric measurement
- **B**iochemical, laboratory results
- **C**linical findings
- **D**ietary recall history

Anthropometric Measurement

Anthropometry is the measurement of body height, weight and proportions.

Other anthropometric measurements

- Mid-arm circumference
- Skin fold thickness
- Head circumference
- Head/chest ratio
- Hip/waist ratio.

Body mass index (BMI) (Table 1)

TABLE 1: WHO classification of BMI

BMI	Assessment
<18.5	Underweight
18.5–24.5	Healthy weight range
25–30	Overweight (grade 1 obesity)
>30–40	Obese (grade 2 obesity)
>40	Very obese (morbid or grade 3 obesity)

Specific Lab Tests

- Measurement of individual nutrient in body fluids (e.g., serum retinol, serum iron, urinary iodine, vitamin D)
- Detect metabolites in the urine (e.g., urinary creatinine/hydroxyl proline ratio).

Clinical Assessment

- It is an essential feature of all nutritional surveys
- It assesses the number of physical signs associated with malnutrition and deficiency of vitamins and micronutrients.
- Good nutritional history should be obtained
- General clinical examination, with special attention to organs such as hair, angles of the mouth, gums, nails, skin, eyes, tongue, muscles, bones and thyroid gland should be done.

Hair

- Spare and thin—Protein, zinc and biotin deficiency
- Easy to pull out—Protein deficiency
- Corkscrew and coiled hair—Vitamin C and A deficiency

Mouth

- Glossitis—Riboflavin, niacin, folic acid, B_{12}
- Bleeding and spongy gums—Vitamin C, A, K, folic acid and niacin
- Angular stomatitis, cheilosis and fissured tongue—B_2, B_6 and niacin
- Leukoplakia—Vitamin A, B_{12}, B-complex, folic acid and niacin
- Sore mouth and tongue—Vitamins B_{12}, B_6, C, niacin, folic acid and iron.

Eyes

- Night blindness, exophthalmia—Vitamin A deficiency
- Photophobia-blurring, conjunctiva inflammation—Vitamins B_2 and A deficiency

Nails

- Spooning—Iron deficiency
- Transverse lines—Protein deficiency

Skin

- Pallor—Folic acid and iron B_2
- Follicular hyperkeratosis—Vitamin B and C
- Flaking dermatitis—PEM, vitamin B_2, vitamin A, zinc and niacin
- Pigmentation and desquamation—Niacin and PEM
- Bruising, purpura—Vitamin K, C and folic acid

Thyroid gland

In mountain areas and areas away from sea, goiter is a reliable sign of iodine deficiency.

Joints and bones

Help detect signs of vitamin D deficiency (rickets) and vitamin C deficiency (scurvy).

Dietary Assessment

It is assessed by five different methods.
- 24-hour dietary recall
- Food frequency questionnaire
- Dietary history since early life
- Food dairy technique
- Observed food consumption.

24-hour dietary recall

- A trained interviewer asks the subject to recall all food and drink taken in the previous 24 hours
- It is quick and easy and depends on short-term memory, but may not be truly representative of the person's usual intake.

Food frequency questionnaire

In this method, the subject is given a list of around 100 food items to indicate his or her intake (frequency and quantity) per day, per week and per month.

Dietary history

- It is an accurate method for assessing the nutritional status
- The information should be collected by a trained interviewer
- Details about usual intake, types, amount, frequency and timing need to be obtained
- Cross-checking the data is important.

Food dairy

- Food intake (types and amounts) should be recorded by the subject at the time of consumption
- The length of the collection period ranges between 1 and 7 days
- Reliable but difficult to maintain.

Observed food consumption

- The meal eaten by the individual is weighed and contents are exactly calculated
- The method is characterized by having a high degree of accuracy but expensive and needs time and efforts.

Assessment of Diet More than 6 Months
Identification data
Child's name ....
Age ....
Sex ....
IP number...
Address ....
Diagnosis...
Relationship with the caregiver/attendant ....

Contd...

Anthropometric measurement

Blood investigation

Clinical diagnosis (physical indicators of nutritional status)

Dietary assessment

- Was the child exclusively breastfeed?
  If yes, the duration_____.
  If no, the nature and mode of artificial feeding_____.
- Does your child take breastfeed now?
  If yes, how many times 24 hours?_____ times.
  Breastfeed during the night?_____ times.
- Any other milk yes/no, If yes, then
  - Which milk_____
  - Amount_____
  - Dilution
  - By katori/spoon/bottle
  - Semi-solid started_____ yes/no?
- At what age semi-solids were started_____ months?
- Child's growth card available: yes/no
  - If available, is the line going well?
  - If not available, what is the child's present weight?
- Is child malnourished?   Yes/No
- In the last week did child eat any
  - Pulses   Yes/No. If yes, how many days_____
  - Dark green vegetables   Yes/No. If yes, how many days_____
  - Eggs/meat/fish   Yes/No. If yes, how many days_____
  - Fruits   Yes/No. If yes, how many days_____
  - Fats and sugars   Yes/No. If yes, how many days_____
- Any difficulty with the child's feeding   Yes/No. If yes, list down _____

Menu Planning

Time	Food items consumed	Amount (g)	Calorie (cal)	Protein (g)
Morning (breakfast)				
Mid-morning (snacks)				
Afternoon (lunch)				
Evening (snacks)				
Dinner				
Pre-sleep (milk/snack)				
Midnight				
	Total			

Evaluation

- Whether the child is getting adequate calories or not:
- Whether the child is getting adequate proteins or not:
- Whether getting all food group items:
- Whether right feeding practices are being followed:
- Decision:
- Action:

Contd...

Assessment of Diet Less than 6 Months

Identification data

Child's name ....

Age ....

Sex ....

IP number ....

Address ....

Diagnosis...

Relationship with the caregiver/attendant ....

Anthropometric measurement

Blood investigation

Clinical diagnosis (physical indicators of nutritional status)

Dietary assessment

- When was the child first fed?
- Whether the baby received any prenatal feeds?_____ Yes/ No
- How many times does breastfeeding given in last 24 hours?
- How many night feeds were given?
- Does the child receive any other food or drink in addition to breastfeed?_____ Yes/ No
  If yes, which food and drink _____
- If animal milk/formula milk_____, how many times in last 24 hours?_____/dilution
- What is being used to feed the child if baby is receiving feed other than breastfeeds?_____(cup/spoon/bottle)
- How feeding bottle/cup is prepared?
  Washing_____ Yes/No
  Boiling _____ Yes/No
- How many times is the baby passing urine in 24 hours?
- Ask the mother if she has much pain during breastfeeding.

BREASTFEEDING

DEFINITION

The method of feeding a baby with milk directly from the mothers, breast is called breastfeeding (Fig. 1).

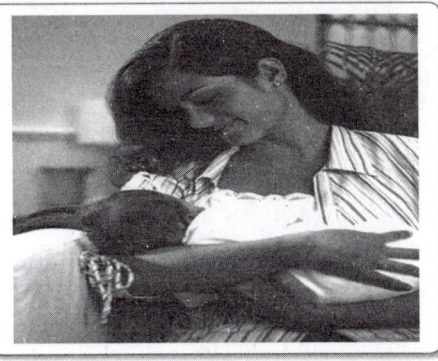

FIG. 1: Method of breastfeeding to the baby

ADVANTAGES OF BREASTFEEDING

Breastfeeding is the safest, cheapest and best protective food for infants. Superiority of human milk is due to its superior nutritive and protective value. It is the perfect food for infants and provides all the nutrient requirements for the first 6 months of life.

Nutritive Value

- Breast milk contains all the nutrients in the right proportion which are needed for optimum growth and development of the baby up to 6 months
- It is essential for the growth of the brain of infants because it has high percentage of lactose and galactose, which are important components of galactocerebroside
- It facilitates absorption of calcium, which helps in bone growth
- It contains amino acids such as taurine and cysteine, which are important as neurotransmitters
- Breast milk fats are polyunsaturated fatty acids which are necessary for the myelination of the nervous system
- It has vitamins, minerals, electrolytes and water in the right proportion for the infants which are necessary for the malnutrition of the intestinal tract.

Digestibility

Breast milk is easily digestible. The proteins of breast milk are mostly lactalbumin and lactoglobulin, which form a soft curd that is easy to digest. The enzyme lipase in the breast milk helps in the digestion of fats and provides free fatty acids.

Protective Value

- Breast milk contains IgA, IgM, macrophages, lymphocytes, unsaturated lactoferrin, lysozyme, complement and interferon
- It also provides protection against malaria and various viral and bacterial infections like skin infections and septicemia
- With exclusive breastfeeding, a baby has fewer chances of developing malnutrition, hypertension, diabetes mellitus, coronary artery disease, arteriosclerosis, ulcerative colitis, appendicitis, etc.

Psychological Benefits

- Breastfeeding promotes close physical and emotional bondage with the mother by frequent skin-to-skin contact, attention and interaction.
- Breastfeeding promotes development of higher intelligence and feeling of security in infants.

Maternal Benefits

- Breastfeeding reduces the chances of postpartum hemorrhage and helps in better uterine involution
- Breastfeeding improves metabolic efficiency and satisfaction with a sense of fulfillments of the mother.

Family and Community Benefits

- Breastfeeding is economical in terms of saving of money, time and energy
- Family has to spend less on milk, health care and illness

- Community expenditure on health care and contraception are reduced. It is economical for the families, hospitals, communities and for countries.

PREPARATION FOR BREASTFEEDING

- Preparation for breastfeeding must be made in the antenatal period
- In the antenatal period, examination of breast and identification of problems such as retracted nipple, should be done with necessary advice for intervention
- In the prenatal period adequate diet should be consumed in terms of energy and nutrients
- Prevention of micronutrient deficiencies, rest, regular exercise, hygienic measures, etc. should be advised for better health in the antenatal period.

INITIATION OF BREASTFEEDING

- Breastfeeding should be initiated within the first half an hour of birth or as soon as possible
- It should also be initiated within one hour even after cesarean section delivery, if the mother and the baby do not have any
- Early suckling provides warmth, security and "colostrum", the baby's first immunization
- Although little in amount, the first milk, colostrum, is most suitable and contains a high concentration of protein and other nutrients needed by baby
- The mother should be made aware of the techniques of breastfeeding. Rooming-in or bedding in should be done with the infant and mother as soon as possible to prevent separation
- No food or drink other than breast milk should be given to the neonates. No water, glucose water, animal milk, gripe or syrup should be given.

INDICATORS OF ADEQUACY OF BREASTFEEDING

Adequacy of breastfeeding is indicated and established by the following:
- Audible swallowing sound during the food
- Let down sensation in mother's breast
- Breast is full before feed and softer afterward
- Wet nappies 6 times in 24 hours
- Frequent soft bowel movement, 3–8 times in 24 hours
- Average weight gain of 18–30 g/day.

DIFFERENT COMPOSITIONS OF BREAST MILK

The composition of breast milk varies at different stages in the postnatal period to fulfill the needs of the baby.

Colostrum

It is secreted during first three days after delivery. It is thick, yellow and less in quantity.

Mature Milk

It is secreted usually from 10 to 12 days after delivery. It is watery but contains all nutrients for optimal growth of the baby.

Preterm Milk

The breast milk secreted by a mother who has delivered a preterm baby is different from milk of a mother who has delivered a full-term baby. This milk contains more proteins, sodium, iron, immunoglobulins and calories appropriate for the requirements of the preterm neonates.

Fore Milk

It is secreted at the starting of the regular breastfeeding. It is more watery to satisfy the baby's thirst and contains more proteins, sugar, vitamins and minerals.

Hind Milk

It is secreted towards the end of regular breastfeeding and contains more fat and energy.

TECHNIQUES OF BREASTFEEDING

- The mother should be comfortable and relaxed physically and mentally before giving breast feed. She should wash her hands and can have a glass of water or milk. She should have no due work in her hands. The baby should be cleaned and dried before feeding, otherwise he/she may feel discomfort and may not cooperate during feeding.
- Correct positioning of the mother and baby is an important aspect of successful breastfeeding. The mother can be lying flat with the infant on top especially following lower uterine cesarean section delivery.

Latching

After proper positioning, when the baby's chin touches the breast, cheek touches the nipple, the baby will open the mouth in 'rooting reflex'.

- Initially, breastfeeding can be given at 1 to 2 hours interval and then on "self-demand" by the baby. A baby usually cries when it feels hungry and then it must be on breastfed.
- Duration of breastfeeding should be continued till the baby is satisfied.
- Burping to be done gently. It is usually not necessary. If the baby is having good latching and attachment during feeding, this would prevent air is form into the baby's mouth.
- Breastfeeding should be continued exclusively up to 4 months of age or preferably may be up to 6 months if adequate breast milk is available.

BREASTFEEDING ASSESSMENT TECHNIQUE

Breastfeeding is the normal way of providing young infants with the nutrients they need for healthy growth and development. According to WHO, exclusive breastfeeding is recommended up to 6 months of age, with continued breastfeeding along with appropriate complementary foods up to 2 years of age or beyond.

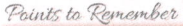
Points to Remember

Benefits of Breastfeeding

The breastfeeding benefits are described as "ABCDEFGH"

Benefits to children:
- A = Allergic diseases conditions are controlled
- B = Best food for children
- C = Close bonding with mother
- D = Development of IQ

Benefits to mother:
- E = Economical
- F = Fitness (mothers returned to pre-pregnancy body shape)
- G = Guard against breast cancer
- H = Hemorrhage reduced (PPH)

***Contraindication of Breastfeeding* to child**
- Galactosemia
- Phenylketonuria (PKU)

To mother (Always ask the mother 'REAL')
- R = Radiotherapy
- E = Ergot therapy
- A = Anti-metabolites therapy
- L = Lithium therapy

Contraindicated Drugs

The contraindicated drugs are described in the form of 'BREAST'
- B—Bromocriptine/benzodiazepines
- R—Radioactive isotopes/rizatriptan
- E—Ergotamine/ethosuximide
- A—Amiodarone/amphetamines
- S—Stimulant laxative/sex hormones
- T—Tetracycline/tretinoin

Breastfeeding Techniques
- Manual breastfeeding techniques
- Breast pump
- Syringe technique

Points to Remember

Observations of Breastfeeding
- Well attachment/poor attachment (follow four steps of good attachment)
- Check position
- Whether the infant's head and body is straight or not?
- Whether the baby is facing breast with the infant's nose opposite her nipple or not?
- Whether the infant's body is close to mother's body or not?
- Whether the mother is supporting the infant's whole body or not?
- Is the infant sucking effectively (that is, slow deep sucks, sometimes pausing)?
- If the baby not sucking effectively or mother complains pain during feeding.
- Check for ulcer in mouth of the baby.
- Check mother's breast for
  - Flat or inverted nipple
  - Engorged breast
  - Breast abscess.

TEN STEPS TO SUCCESSFUL BREASTFEEDING

Step 1: Have a return breastfeeding policy that is routinely communicated to all health staff.

Step 2: Train whole health care staff in skills necessary to implement this policy. The training should include:

- Advantages of breastfeeding
- Risk of artificial feeding and use of bottles
- Mechanism of lactation and sucking
- How to help mothers initiate and sustain breastfeeding
- How to assess a breastfeeding session
- How to resolve breastfeeding difficulties
- Orientation and education on hospital
- Importance of feeding on cue
- Positioning and attachment

Step 3: Inform all pregnant women about the benefits and management of breastfeeding

Step 4: Help mothers initiate breastfeeding within half an hour after childbirth.

- Place the babies in skin-to-skin contact with their mothers immediately following birth for at least an hour and encourage mother to recognize when their babies are ready to breastfeed, offering help if needed.

Step 5: Show mothers how to breastfeed and how to maintain lactation, even if they are separated from their infants.

Step 6: Give newborns no food or drink other than breast milk, not even sips of water, unless medically indicated.

- No promotion of infant foods/drinks should be done and there should be acceptable medical reasons for supplementation like.
- Infant condition
  - Sucking difficulties or oral abnormalities
  - Very low birthweight or preterm infants
  - Infants at risk of hypoglycemia, dehydrated or malnourished
- Maternal conditions
  - Mother is on antithyroid medications
  - Mother has breast abscess
  - Avoidance of all breastfeed by HIV +ve mothers is recommended when replacement feeding is acceptable, feasible, affordable, sustainable and safe.
  - Breastfeed is not encouraged for a mother with human T-cell leukemia virus.

Step 7: Practice rooming in, that is, allow mothers and infants to remain together 24 hours a day. Benefits of rooming-in are as follows.

- Reduces cost
- Requires minimal equipment
- Reduces infection
- Helps in establishing and maintaining breastfeeding
- Facilitates the bonding process

Step 8: Encourage breastfeeding on demand. Breastfeed on demand results in:

- Earlier passage of meconium
- Lower maximal weight loss

- Breast milk flow is established sooner
- Larger volume of milk intake from day 3
- Fewer incidents of jaundice
- Prevents engorgement of breast

Step 9: Give no artificial teats or pacifiers (also called dummies or soothers) to breastfeeding infants. Alternatives to artificial teats are as follows:

- Cup
- Spoon
- Dropper
- Syringe

Step 10: Foster the establishment of breastfeeding support groups and refer mothers to them on discharge from the hospital or clinic.

- Support group can include
  - Early postnatal or clinic checkup
  - Home visit
  - Telephone calls
  - Community services
  - Outpatient breastfeeding clinics

FORMULA PREPARATION AND ARTIFICIAL FEEDING

PREPARATION OF FORMULA

The most commonly recommended milk for formula feeding is cow's milk.

Articles Needed

- A wide mouth straight bottle and teats
- Large pan with cover for boiling equipment
- Measuring cup
- Measuring tablespoon and teaspoon
- Pan with cover for boiling bottles and nipples
- Tong's bottle brush
- Small jar with tight lid for storing nipples
- Long handled spoon
- Large jug
- Table knife

Procedure

- Equipment is washed with hot, soapy water.
- Inside of the bottle is cleaned with a bottle brush.
- Nipples are rubbed inside and outside with table salt, and water is squeezed out through the holes.
- All the equipment except rubber articles are placed in a covered container and boiled for 10–15 minutes.

- Nipples and rubber caps are boiled for 3 minutes only.
- Water is boiled in a tea kettle or a pan and required amount is transferred to a jug using a sterile measure.
- A measured amount of sugar and milk is transferred to the jug.
- The formula is stirred thoroughly and poured in sterile feeding bottles.
- Bottles are covered with bottle caps and placed in a pan of cold water to cool quickly.
- The bottles are then transferred to the refrigerator, the cap is replaced with a nipple and the bottle is placed in warm water.
- If refrigerator facilities are not available, the formula is prepared fresh at every feed.
- Bottles and nipples can be boiled once or twice a day and kept covered for use.
- Hands should be thoroughly washed before handling milk or the bottle.

FEEDING SCHEDULE

- Baby is offered first feed by 4–6 hours
- Diluted cow's milk (2:1) with added sugar (1 teaspoonful (TSF) per 100 mL) during first 2 weeks.
- Diluted milk (3:1) with sugar (1/2 TSF per 100 mL) during next 2–4 weeks followed by undiluted cow's milk with or without sugar is offered every 3–4 hours (2–3 hours for small infants).
- Gradually the feeding interval is increased as in breastfeeding.
- Amount of milk taken at each feed varies. There is no rule of thumb. It is preferable to offer 15 mL in next feed if the baby completely empties the bottle.

Table 2 shows an approximate guide

TABLE 2: **Amount of the feeds as per the age**

Age	Amount of feed (mL)
1st week	50
2nd week	75
3rd week to 2 months	100–150
2–3 months	150–175
3–4 months	175–200
5–12 months	200–250

DAILY REQUIREMENTS OF MILK

Calculations are based on the child's daily caloric needs of 110–120 kcal and fluids 150 mL per kg during early months.

Example

- Daily requirements of a 2-month-old baby weighing 4 kg
- Calories: $4 \times (110–120) = 400–480$ kcal
- Fluids: $4 \times 150 = 600$ mL
- If undiluted cow's milk is used, then 600 mL of milk will provide $600 \times 67/100 = 402$ kcal
- Sugar: 3 TSF (1/2 TSF/100 mL) = $3 \times 16 = 48$ kcal
- Total calories = $402 + 48 = 450$ kcal

- If diluted cow's milk is used, sugar may be increased up to 1 TSF per 100 mL
- In hot weather, fluid needs are much higher (up to 200 mL/kg)

ARTIFICIAL FEEDING

Definition

Artificial feeding is a form of complementary or substituted feeding given to a baby instead of breastfeeding.

Indications

- Insufficient breast milk
- Death of the mother
- Working mother
- Pregnancy
- Diseases of the breast
- Infectious diseases to the mother (e.g., TB, HIV)
- Chronic diseases (e.g., heart and kidney diseases)
- Mental illness
- A child with poor sucking reflex, e.g. prematurity, birth trauma etc.

Articles Needed

A sterile vessel containing:
- Bottle
- Teat
- Cap
- Rim
- Cups with lid and paladai
- Strainer
- Ounce glass
- Spoon

A clean tray containing:
- Duster
- Transferring forceps
- Boiled cooled water in a kettle
- Sugar
- A jug with milk or prescribed formula tin
- Sauce pan with lid to boil milk
- Big bowl with water to cool the milk
- Bib
- Draw sheet and mackintosh
- Gown

Procedure

- Check the doctor's order and do the calculation accordingly

- Collect the necessary equipment
- Wash hands with soap and water
- Measure the required amount of water and milk and pour in the sauce pan
- Add one teaspoon of sugar to 90 mL of liquid
- Boil the milk until it reaches boiling point
- Cool the milk in the bowl of water till it is warm enough for the child to drink
- Strain the milk into a cup
- Pour into feeding bottle
- Wash hands and wear gown
- Make sure that the baby is dry and clean
- Place a mackintosh and a draw sheet of cloth under the infant as a result of gastrocolic reflex that is stimulated by feeding
- Mummify the infant if needed
- Put towel or bib under the chin to prevent the soiling of infant's dress
- The nurse or the mother should sit comfortably on a chair with legs crossed
- Test the temperature of the milk and rate of flow
- Place the entire nipple tip in the infant's mouth
- Bottle should be held in upright position throughout the feeding to prevent entry of air
- The nipple should always be filled with milk; otherwise the infant will suck in air
- In between and after feeding, the baby should be burped and cuddled
- Place the baby in bed in right lateral position to facilitate gastric emptying
- Wash and replace the articles

KATORI AND SPOON FEEDING/PALADAI FEEDING

Introduction

Feeding with a spoon and katori has been found to be safe in small for gestational age.

Indications

- Small for gestational age infants
- Premature babies who have good swallowing reflex but poor sucking reflex.

Advantages

- This mode of feeding is a bridge between gavage feeding and direct breastfeeding.
- Chances for transmission of infection associated with feeding is less when compare to bottle feeding.
- Best method for stable premature and low birthweight infants.

Disadvantages

- Cannot replace direct breastfeeding advantages
- Delay in development of sucking reflex

Articles Needed

A sterile tray containing

- Sterilized bowl
- Small spoon/paladai
- Expressed breast milk in a glass
- Face towel
- Bib
- Sterile oral syringe

Preparation

- Explain the mother why we need to feed through spoon or paladai
- Assist the mother in expression of breast milk
- Check the neonatologist's order for feeding amount, frequency and any other precautions
  - Wipe the face of the baby with towel
  - Perform hand hygiene
  - Measure the required amount of feed and pour into a katori
  - Wear the bib around the child's neck
  - Make the mother to sit comfortably. The head of the baby should be held at crook of arm of the mother. Ask the mother to support the baby's body with the side of hand.
  - Take the milk from katori with the help of the spoon
  - Place the spoon or spike of the paladai at the corner of the mouth and milk should be allowed to flow into the infants mouth slowly, avoiding any spillage
- This process should be repeated till the required amount has been fed.

Post Procedure Care

- Remove bib from the neck.
- Burp the child as explained in breastfeeding
- Document the procedure in nurses record with time, amount of feed, any observations made during feeding.

COMPLEMENTARY FEEDING

Definition

Complementary feeding is the process of giving other foods and liquids with breast milk after the age of 6 months.

Points to Remember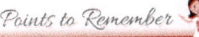

- Wash hands
- Keep food in clean utensils
- Cook food thoroughly
- Keep food at safe temperature
- Meet the nutritional requirements of the child
- Locally available, seasonable food must be given
- Gradually increase the quantity of food to the child
- Use safe water
- Give freshly prepared food to baby
- Keep the cooked food covered

Types of Complementary Food

- Pure liquids: Dal soup, vegetable soup, rice water and fruit juices.
- Semi-liquids: Chopped vegetables, pulses.
- Semisolids: Mashed potatoes, pulses boiled vegetables, mashed banana, soft cooked rice and fish.
- Solids: Cooked rice, chapati, bread, biscuits, groundnuts, banana, apple and seasonal fruits.

Quantity and Frequency of Complementary Food for Children

- 2–3 times a day for 6–8 months and energy required is 200 kcal/day
- 3–4 times a day for 9–11 months and energy required is 300 kcal/day and
- 3–4 times a day for 12–23 months and energy required is 550 kcal/day.

Problems

- Diarrhea
- Malnutrition
- Abdominal pain
- Indigestion

Feeding of Older Children

- To establish good dietary habits, the child should be served meals at regular intervals
- Food should be attractive and digestible for his age
- Provide adequate time at meals
- Above all, diet must be balanced and the baby should be provided adequate amounts of proteins for growth, fats and carbohydrates for energy needs and vitamins and minerals.

FOOD GROUP	
Daily Requirements/Servings Per Day	
• Milk and cheese	– 500 mL milk/equivalent
• Protein group:	
▪ Egg	– one
▪ Meat and fish etc.	– one serving
▪ Beans, peas etc.	– one serving
• Vegetable and fruit group	
▪ Vitamin C group (citrus fruits, tomato etc.)	equivalent to one orange (one citrus fruit = double the weight of tomato)
▪ Vitamin A group (green or yellow vegetables and fruits) one serving	
▪ Other vegetables and fruits	one serving each
• Cereal group (bread, chapatti etc.)	3–4 servings
• Fat group (butter, ghee, oils)	20–40 g
• Sugar, jaggery etc.	40–50 g

RECOMMENDED DAILY DIETARY ALLOWANCES (TABLES 3 AND 4)

TABLE 3: Recommended daily dietary allowances

Nutrient	Under 1 Year	1–6 Years	Over 6 Years
Water (mL/kg)	125–150	100–125	50–100
Calories (per kg)	100–120	80–100	50–80
Protein g/kg	2.5–3.5	2.0–2.5	1.0–2.0
Iron (mg)	10.0	15.0	20.0
Calcium (g)	0.5	1.0	1.5
Vitamin A (IU)	1500	2500	5000
Vitamin D (IU)	400	400	800
Vitamin C (mg)	30	10	50
Thiamine (mg)	0.5	1.0	1.5
Riboflavin (mg)	0.5	1.0	1.5
Nicotinic acid (mg)	6.0	12.0	18.0
Pyridoxine (mg)	0.5	1.0	1.5
B12 (mg)	0.2	0.5	1.0
Folic acid (ug)	25	50	100

TABLE 4: Various vegetable proteins which can be added to a child's diet

Food stuff	Protein (g/100 g)
Bengal gram	17.0
Bengal gram roasted	22.0
Lentil	20
Peas	25.0
Rajmah	33.0
Soybeans	43.0
Field beans	25.0
Groundnut cake	40.0
Groundnut	25.0

MALNUTRITION ASSESSMENT (TABLES 5 TO 8)

Formula for calculating the degree of malnutrion

$$\text{Degree of malnutrition} = \frac{\text{Actual weight of the child}}{\text{Expected weight of the child}} \times 100$$

TABLE 5: Classification of nutritional status (welcome trust classification)

Nutritional status	Expected weight for age	Presence of edema
Normal	More than 80%	No
Undernutrition	60–80%	No
Kwashiorkar	60–80%	Yes
Marasmus	Less than 60%	No
Marasmus and kwashiorkar	Less than 60%	Yes

TABLE 6: **Degree of malnutrition**

Percentage of malnutrition	Degree of malnutrition
90–95	Normal
75–85	First
65–75	Second
<65	Third

TABLE 7: **IAP classification based on weight for age**

80–100%	Normal
71–80%	Grade I
61–70%	Grade II
51–60%	Grade III
<50%	Grade IV

TABLE 8: **WHO classification of malnutrition**

Weight for height	Height for age	Label
>80%	>90%	Normal
>80%	<90%	Stunted
<80%	>90%	Wasted
<80%	<90%	Wasted and stunted growth

Methods of Feeding

- ⇒ Gastrostomy Feeding
- ⇒ Gavage Feeding/Nasogastric Feeding
- ⇒ Total Parenteral Nutrition
- ⇒ Infusion Pump
- ⇒ Jejunostomy and Enterostomy Feeding

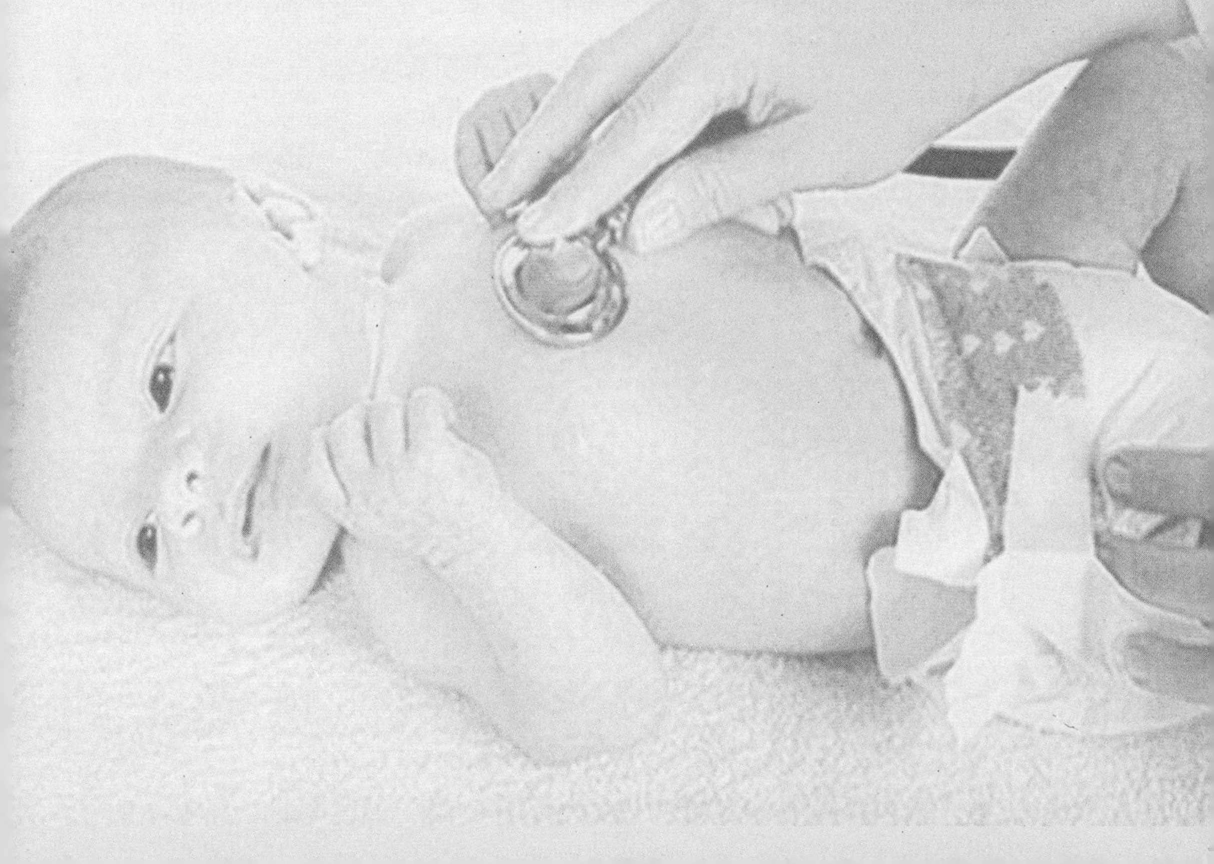

LEARNING OBJECTIVES

On the completion of this chapter, the pediatric nurse will be able to perform the following activities:
- Define gastrostomy feeding.
- Develop skills in gastrostomy feeding
- Define gavage feeding
- List the purpose and explain the procedure in detail
- Develop skills in gavage feeding
- Compare with checklist to maintain standard performance
- Define Jejunostomy and enterostomy
- Explain the techniques and purpose of feeding
- Develop skills in this procedure
- Inculcate the practice in their field

GASTROSTOMY FEEDING

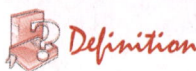 Definition

Gastrostomy feeding is a means of providing nourishment and fluids via a tube that has been surgically inserted via a stab wound through the abdominal wall into the stoma.

PURPOSES

- To provide a method for nutrition and fluids that requires minimal effort when the patient is unable to suck or swallow for long periods of time.
- To allow for better decompression of stomach (because of large tube size).
- To provide a safe method of feeding a child with esophageal stricture or one who cannot tolerate alternative method.
- To provide a route that allows adequate kilo joule (calorie) and/or fluid intake in a child with chronic lung disease or in one who does not have continuity of the gastrointestinal tract, i.e., esophageal atresia.

ARTICLES NEEDED

- Warm feeding fluid at 38°C
- Dummy
- Reservoir syringe or tunnel
- Syringe for aspirating.

PREPARATORY PHASE

- Gastrostomy tube should be in 1 of 3 positions between feedings
  - Lowered and open to start drainage.
  - Open, connected to reservoir (funnel and syringe), i.e. elevated 10–12 cm.
  - Clamped
  - Figure 1 shows Gastrostomy feeding

PROCEDURE

Steps	Rationale
• The nurse may be directed to check residual stomach contents prior to feeding	This is done to monitor the appropriate fluid intake, digestion time and overfeeding that can cause distension
• Attach syringe and aspirate stomach contents	Residual fluid may be returned to stomach or discarded depending on amount
• A Y-tube which is connected at the point where reservoir and gastrostomy tube join may be used during feeding	To provide simultaneous decompression during feeding
• When feeding is about to begin, the infant should be placed in comfortable position in bed either flat or with head slightly elevated. If condition permits, the nurse should hold the infant. A dummy can be given	When the infant is comfortable and relaxed, feeding fluid will flow more easily in the stomach. A dummy will satisfy normal sucking activity, provide exercise for jaw, muscles and relax musculature as well as provide pleasure normally associated with feeding
• Attach a reservoir syringe to tube (if not already open to continuous elevation) and fill prior to unclamping tube	Prevents air from entering tube (and then stomach), which may cause distension
• Elevate tube and reservoir to 10–12 cm above the abdominal wall. Do not apply any pressure to start the flow	This elevation level will allow for slow, gravity-induced flow pressure, which may cause a flow of fluid back into the esophagus
• Feed slowly, taking 20–45 minutes. Fill reservoir with remaining fluid before it is empty to avoid instillation of air	A rapid feeding will interfere with normal peristalsis and will cause abdominal distension and back flow into the reservoir or oesophagus
• Continue to provide the infant with pleasant feeling associated with feeding	This rinses tubing and will prevent clogging
• When feeding is completed: Clear water to be instilled (10–30 mL) if tube is to be clamped. Apply clamp before water level reaches end of the reservoir	Skin breakdown is caused by continued exposure to stomach contents that may be leaking out around tube constant pulling on the tube can cause widening of skin opening and subsequent leakage
• Check dressing and skin around the point for tube entry for wetness. Clean skin and apply skin barrier preparation or ointment. See that there is no pull on the tube	To promote relaxation and improved digestion of feeding
• Leave the infant dry and comfortable. If unable to hold him during feeding, this may be a good time to fondle and provide him with warmth and love	Documentation
• Accurately describe and record procedure, including time of feeding, fluid given, amount and characteristic of residual (if any) and what was done with it, how the patient tolerated feeding, any abdominal distension	

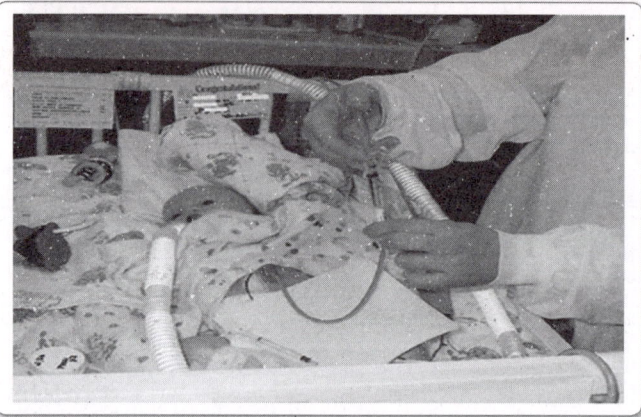

FIG. 1: Gastrostomy feeding

GAVAGE FEEDING/NASOGASTRIC FEEDING

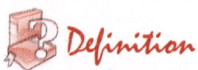 Definition

Gavage feeding is an artificial method of giving fluids and nutrients. This is a process of feeding with the tube (nasogastric tube) inserted through the nose, pharynx, esophagus and into the stomach.

PURPOSES AND INDICATIONS

- To feed the children who are unable to take feed orally.
- Feed the children who are undergoing oral surgery such as cleft lip or cleft palate, fracture of jaw, and has difficulty in swallowing.
- When the patient is unconscious or semiconscious.
- When the condition is not supportive to take large amount of food orally, e.g. severe burns, malnutrition, prematurity, acute and chronic infections.
- Conditions when the patient is unable to retain the food, e.g. anorexia nervosa and vomiting.

ADVANTAGES OF NASOGASTRIC FEEDING

- All types of nutrients including distasteful foods and medications can be given in adequate amount.
- Without any danger, feeding can be continued for weeks.
- According to need, stomach can be aspirated at any time.
- Large amount of fluids can be given with safety.

ARTICLES NEEDED

- Mackintosh with towel
- Kidney tray for receiving the waste
- Cotton tipped applicators to clean the nostrils

- Ryle's tube in a bowel
- Lubricants such as water soluble jelly on glycerin to prevent friction
- Gauze pieces to clean the secretions
- Scissors and adhesive plaster or tape
- Measuring cup or glass/ounces glass
- Sterile syringe, about 10–20 mL
- Paper bag to collect the wastes
- Glass of feed in a bowel of warm water to give the feed at the body temperature
- Tongue blade
- Suction apparatus—to clear the airway, whenever need
- Bowel with water—to test the location of tube
- Clamp—to clamp the tube to prevent leakage of gastric contents.

PROCEDURE

- Identify the patient.
- Explain the procedure to the patient.
- Maintain privacy.
- Make the patient in comfortable position.
- Make the patient sit on chair or place him in Fowler's position.
- Arrange the mackintosh and face towel across the chest and put under the chin to protect the garments and bed linens.
- Keep the kidney tray ready for receiving the vomit, if it occurs.
- Remove the dentures and place in a bowl of clean water.
- Clean the nostrils with cotton applicators, if secretions are deposited.
- Arrange all articles near the bedside or on the bedside locker.
- Wash hands properly.
- Check the patency of the tube.
- Measure the length of the tube by measuring it from the tip of the nose to earlobe and from earlobe to the tip of the xiphoid process of the sternum.
- Wear hand gloves.
- Lubricate the tube with glycerin or jelly by the piece of gauze. It starts from tip to the 6–8 inches long.
- Now slowly insert the tube with the right hand into the left nostril.
- Pass the tube slowly backward and the patient downward. When the tube reaches at pharynx, give the patient sips of water to swallow, while swallows; insert the tube about 3–4 inches each time. Insert it till the mark stop to insert appears.
- Now confirm the placement of the tube by aspirating the gastric contents with the syringe. Other method is to place the tube end in a bowl of water and check the bubbles. If bubbles are present, it indicates position in trachea.
- Examine the mouth of the patient with tongue blade and a light source.
- Then, secure the tube with the adhesive tape at the nasal bridge.
- After some time, give some water to the patient to expel the air. Give the feed with feeding syringe or funnel. Give feed slowly; do not push the feeding solution with a plunger.

- When the feeding is completed, pour a little amount of water and clamp the tube firmly to prevent leakage of fluids.
- When any obstruction occurs while feeding, remove the funnel and take a syringe with sterile water. Push the water slowly, and draw it back from gastric contents. When fluid starts to enter, connect the feeding funnel with tube.
- Provide oral hygiene every 4–6 hours to prevent infections.
- Dispose the waste materials and clean the articles properly and replace them.
- Do the hand washing.
- Recording and reporting.
- Figure 2 shows the nasogastric tube feeding in a child.

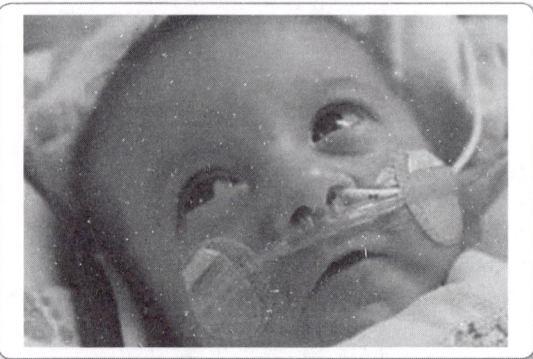

FIG. 2: Nasogastric tube feeding

TOTAL PARENTERAL NUTRITION

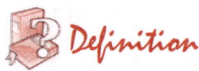 *Definition*

Total parenteral nutrition (TPN) is an intravenous (IV) nutrition. TPN solution will provide your child with all or most of his or her calories and nutrients.

According to Jane Anne Yaworski, MSN, RN, a Clinical Nurse Specialist in the Nutrition Support Service and Intestinal Care Center, "parenteral" actually means to eat (-enteral) through an IV (par-).

INDICATIONS

- Gastrointestinal (GI) disorder that severely limits the ability of a patient's digestive tract.
- Short bowel syndrome commonly known as short gut syndrome.
- The condition in which most of the small intestine is either missing or does not work.
- Malnourished and failure to thrive.
- Nutritional requirement before surgery.
- With prolonged postoperative complications
- With inadequate oral intake
- Preterm newborns.

PURPOSES

- To get nutrition for growth and development
- To maintain water and electrolyte balance.

TYPE OF SOLUTIONS

Protein, carbohydrates (in the form of glucose), glucose, fat, vitamins and mineral.

METHODS OF TPN ADMINISTRATION

- Continuous administration over 24 hours period
- Cyclic basis over a 12 hours period during night.

TYPES OF VENOUS ACCESS DEVICES

- Groshong catheter
- Tunneled catheter
- Implanted ports totally implantable metal or plastic device.

NURSE'S RESPONSIBILITY IN ADMINISTERING TOTAL PARENTERAL NUTRITION

- Before starting TPN, the nurse needs to assess the nutritional status and physical growth in children below 3 years, including head circumference, for comparison of information to monitor the response of the child to TPN.
- Review indication of TPN.
- Determine the baseline vital signs and activity level, hydration status, venous access route as central or peripheral.
- Assemble and prepare equipment and supplies as needed.
- Administer TPN using strict aseptic technique—the preliminary steps include:
  - Connect tubing, filter and Y connections.
  - Connect tubing, to solutions and prime tubing with solution.
  - Insert tubing into infusion pump and set flow rate.
- Verify the patency of venous access and check the site hourly for signs of infiltration.
- Monitor vital signs activity level at 4 hours.
- Monitor the intake and output.

COMPLICATIONS

- Infection
- Liver disease and damage
- Growth and developmental delays
- Hyperglycemia
- Electrolyte imbalance
- Dehydration
- Air embolism

INFUSION PUMP

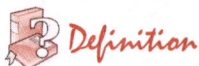 *Definition*

Infusion pump is a medical device through which the nutrients and medications such as insulin or other hormones, antibiotics, chemotherapy drugs and analgesics are infused into the patient's body at steady rates.

TYPES OF INFUSION

- Continuous infusion—consists of small pulses of infusion between 500 nanoliters and 10 m^2.
- Intermittent infusion—has a 'high' infusion rate, alternating with a low infusion rate to keep the cannula open. This mode is often used to administer antibiotics and other drugs that can irritate a blood vessel.
- Patient-controlled—infusion on-demand. The rate is controlled by a pressure pad or a button that can be activated by the patient. Repeated small doses of opioid analgesia are delivered. Total parenteral nutrition usually requires an infusion curve similar to normal meal times.
- Figure 3 shows a Baxter International CX infusion pump

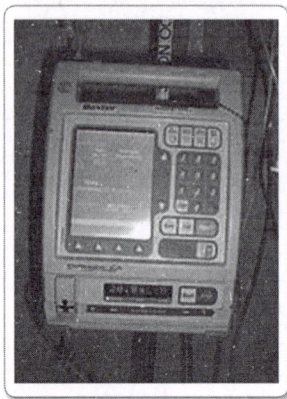

FIG. 3: A Baxter International Colleague CX infusion pump

CLASSES OF PUMPS

- There are two basic classes of pumps:
    - Large-volume pumps: These can pump nutrient solutions large enough to feed a patient.
    - Small-volume pumps: These infuse hormone such as insulin or other medicines, such as opiates.
- Anti-free-flow devices prevent blood from draining from the patient or infuse from freely entering the patient, when the infusion pump is being set up.
- A 'down pressure' sensor will detect when the patient's vein is blocked, or the line to the patient is kinked. This may be configurable for high (subcutaneous and epidural) or low (venous) applications.
- **An 'air-in-line' detector:** A typical detector that will use an ultrasonic transmitter and receiver to detect when air is being pumped. Some pumps actually measure the volume and may even have configurable volumes, from 0.1 to 2 mL of air. None of these amounts can cause harm, but sometimes the air can interfere with the infusion of a low-dose medicine.

- An 'up pressure' sensor can detect when the bag or syringe is empty, or even if the bag or syringe is being squeezed.
- A drug library with customizable programmable limits for individual drugs is needed that helps to avoid medication errors.
- Mechanisms to avoid uncontrolled flow of drugs in large volume pumps.
- Many pumps include an internal electronic log of the last several thousand therapy events. These are usually tagged with the time and date from the pump's clock. Usually, erasing the log is a feature protected by a security code, specifically to detect staff abuse of the pump or patient.
- Many models of infusion pump can be configured to display only a small subset of features while they are operating, in order to prevent tampering by patients, untrained staff and visitors.
- Using a volumetric IV **pump, calculate** the duration of 1,000 mL of normal saline being **infused** at 125 mL/hour.
- There are 250 mL of D$_5$W being **infused** at 33 gtt/min on IV tubing calibrated at 10 gtt/mL. **Calculate the infusion**

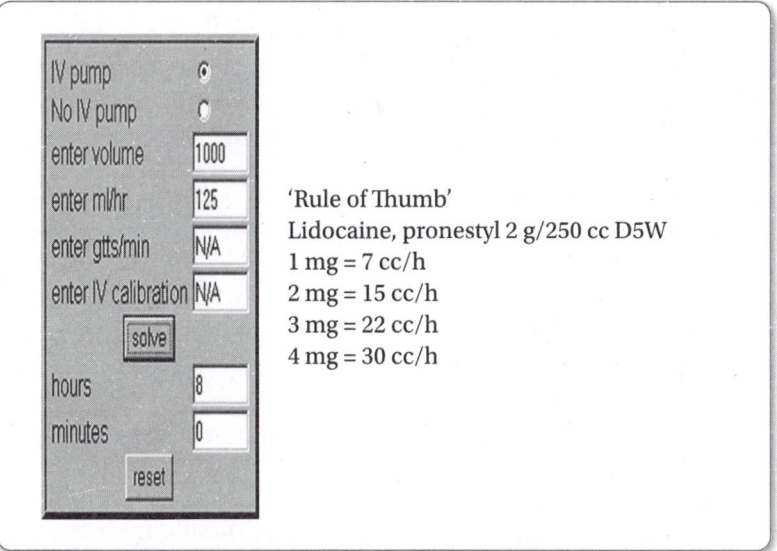

'Rule of Thumb'
Lidocaine, pronestyl 2 g/250 cc D5W
1 mg = 7 cc/h
2 mg = 15 cc/h
3 mg = 22 cc/h
4 mg = 30 cc/h

FIG. 4: Calculate the infusion

JEJUNOSTOMY AND ENTEROSTOMY FEEDING

JEJUNOSTOMY

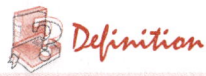 *Definition*

Jejunostomy is a surgical procedure by which a tube is put in the lumen of the proximal jejunum primarily to administer nutrition.

ENTEROSTOMY

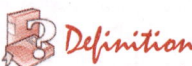 Definition

An enterostomy is an operation in which the surgeon makes a passage into the small intestine through the abdomen with an opening to allow for drainage or to insert a tube for feeding.

TECHNIQUE

- Open jejunostomy
- Needle catheter technique
- Percutaneous endoscopy
- Laparoscopy

PURPOSE

Nutrition can be influenced at the level of jejunum:
- To protect a surface lying in the stomach which has leaked.
- To protect a surface lying in the duodenum following an injury.
- Healing an inflamed bowel segment.
- Enterostomy is needed to prevent the contest of the intestine from causing serious inflammation inside the abdominal cavity.
- An esophageal obstruction which is correctable. Irrespective of the pathology or surgical procedure of the esophagus, stomach and duodenum.

PLACEMENT OF A TUBE FOR EXTERNAL FEEDING

- External feeding is a method for covering nutritional solution directly in to the stomach or jejunum through a tube.
- Tube enterostomies may be long term but not permanent.
- Enterostomy is usually performed only as emergency treatment for traumatic injuries in the abdomen.

ARTICLES NEEDED

- Tube to be used
- Foil bowl
- Universal indicator paper with color chart
- 500 mL syringe
- Tape suitable for the condition of the child skin

PROCEDURE

- Make a small laparotomy incision in the upper abdomen under local or general anesthesia.
- Find the upper jejunum of the patient by following it downward from the duodenojejunal flexure.
- Confirm that it is his/her duodenojejunal junction by finding his inferior mesenteric vein along his left border.

- It emerges from its fixed position behind his peritoneum.
- Take a loop from his duodenojejunal junction and make an incision on its anterior enteric border through the longitudinal muscle layer.
- Insert a feeding catheter or long Ryle's tube through this hole.
- Make a second incision in his abdominal wall above where this loop of jejunum comfortably lies.
- Draw the end of the tube back through his abdominal wall.
- Close the abdomen and anchor the tube to his abdominal wall with a Saxon stocking type of anchoring stitch or with tape.

NURSING RESPONSIBILITY IN JEJUNOSTOMY AND ENTEROSTOMY

- The position of the tube is checked to see whether it is properly placed or not.
- Attach the syringe to the tubing.
- Attach the syringe to the catheter and pour a small amount of feeding into it.
- Elevate the syringe above the mattress.
- Before the syringe is empty, pinch the tubing with fingers to prevent air entering.
- The rate of the flow depends on the height of the syringe on the diameter of the tubing.
- The feeding should flow slowly to prevent regurgitation.
- Follow the feeding with a small amount of water to flush the tubing.
- If the catheter is to be left in place, it should be capped or clamped to prevent the entrance of air.
- Care of the skin around the jejunostomy is exceedingly important to prevent irritation and infection.
- The area is kept clean and covered with a sterile dressing.
- The dressing must be changed as frequently as necessary to keep the area clean and dry.
- Ointment or other preparation may be prescribed to be used daily or as necessary as an aid to healing.
- After the wound healing, a dressing may not be necessary.
- When the child no longer needs the jejunostomy, the tube is removed and the abdominal opening closes and contracts spontaneously.

COMPLICATIONS

- Infection gastrointestinal tract
- Tube dislocation
- Obstruction or migration of the tube
- Intra-abdominal abscess
- Enterocutaneous fistula
- Abdominal distension
- Constipation

AFTER CARE

- Monitoring the surgical wound for infection or bleeding.
- Leading to keep stoma clean.
- Patient's fluid intake and output will be checked frequency to minimize the risk of hydration.

7

Instillation of Medications

LEARNING OBJECTIVES

On the completion of this chapter, the pediatric nurse will be able to perform the following activities:
- Explain the techniques and purpose of instillation of medication into eyes, ear and nose
- Develop skill in this procedure
- Inculcate the skills in their practical field.
- Explain the techniques and purposes of injections
- Develop skill in this procedure
- Inculcate the skills in their practical field.

Instillation of medications involves—medications into the eye, ear and nose. A slight abnormal deviation during the medication can cause a vast impact on the organ.

EYE

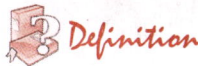 *Definition*

Administer the medication into the eyes by using aseptic, safety technique for various therapeutic purposes.

PURPOSES FOR EYE MEDICATION

- To lubricate the eyes.
- For the management of infections.
- For examination of eye before surgical procedure.
- For finding the abrasions and scars in the cornea by staining with medications.
- To clean the eyes from dust.
- To keep the eyes healthy and maintain the visualization by safety precautions.
- To dilate, constrict pupil and local anesthesia to eye.

ARTICLES NEEDED

- A set of disposable gloves for wearing (optional) in hands to prevent contamination.
- Prescribed medication by the physician.
- Six to eight dry cotton balls.
- Cotton balls soaked in normal saline.
- Sterile dry dressing pad.
- Paper bag or kidney tray for discarding the waste.

Points to Remember

- Instillation of medication involves good care, good skill, adequate position, adequate amount of medication and sterile techniques.
- Do the proper identification of the patient and match with the record.
- Check the medication as per the physician's order, number of drops and side of eye for the treatment.
- Check the medication for manufacturing date and expiry.
- Assess the child for any allergy to medications.
- Explain the child about the procedure, especially to older children.
- Provide the comfortable position—supine position with head should be slightly hyperextended.
- Provide restraint (mummy) if needed.

PROCEDURE OF EYE DROP INSTILLATION (FIG. 1)

- The nurse should wash the hands and wear the gloves.
- Clean the eyes with sterile normal saline soaked cotton swab from inner canthus to outer canthus.
- Advise the child to look up to the ceiling.
- The nurse should fill the dropper and stand behind the child's head.
- Expose the lower conjunctival sac by placing the thumb and finger of left hand at lower margin of the eyelid and pressing downwards gently towards the cheek.
- The medication drops should be instilled onto the outer third of lower conjunctival sac at prescribed number of drops. The medication should be instilled on the conjunctival sac, not directly on the cornea. The first drop of medication should be discarded.
- While instillation of medication, the dropper should be hold 1–2 cm above the eye.

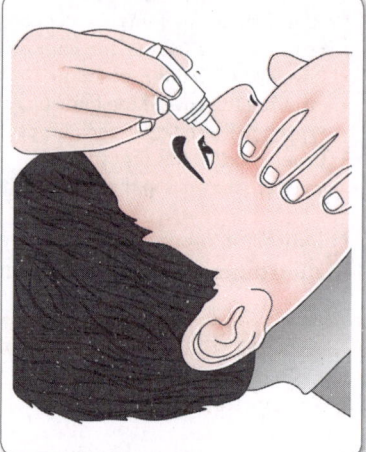

FIG. 1: Instillation of medication into the eye

APPLICATION OF EYE OINTMENT

- First clean the nozzle of the tube with the dry sterile cotton swab.
- The first bead of ointment should be discarded.
- Squeeze the tube and apply thin strip of ointment on the lower conjunctival sac (exposed fornix) from inner canthus to outward.
- Extra medication should be wiped with cotton swab.
- After medication, advise the child to close the eyes and not to squeeze, as to prevent the injury and push out medication.
- Eyelids should be cleaned with sterile cotton swab from inner canthus to outer canthus.
- If needed, then apply the dressing pad and cover them with a tape.
- Replace all the articles and wash the hands.
- Do the recording and reporting.
- Do the assessment of the child.
- Observe for response and complications.
- When more than one medication are prescribed, then at least 5–7 minutes interval should be followed after administration of one medication.

EAR

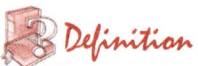 *Definition*

Administration of medication into the ears for various therapeutic purposes by using safe and hygienic techniques.

PURPOSES FOR EAR MEDICATIONS

- To reduce the inflammation and pain.
- To inhibit the growth and destroy the harmful microorganisms in the ear canal.

- To help in the removal of foreign bodies from the ear canal.
- To remove the earwax by making it soft.
- To maintain the antibacterial or anti-microorganism effect in ear canal and keep it free from any infections.

ARTICLES NEEDED

- Medication bottle with the clean sterile dropper.
- Cotton-tipped applicators.
- Cotton balls.
- Bowel with normal saline (if needed).
- Kidney tray or paper bag.
- Sterile disposable gloves (optional).
- Recording, reporting articles.

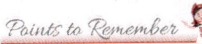
Points to Remember

- Identify the correct patient.
- Check the medications—name, date of manufacturing, expiry date, dose and allergy to medications.
- Do not instill hydrocortisone ear drops in case of a child with fungal or viral infections.

PROCEDURE

- Explain the procedure to gain the cooperation.
- Provide the sidelying position and keep the ear to be treated uppermost.
- If necessary, provide the restraint (mummy restraint) to the child.
- Clean the meatus of the ear canal with the help of cotton-tipped applicators; if necessary, use the normal saline.
- First warm the container of medication by keeping it in the hand or by placing it in warm water for short time to prevent chilling sensation, nausea and vertigo.
- Fill the dropper with medication.
- Make the auditory canal straight, if the child is under 3 years of age, pull the pinna down and backward. It the child is more than 3 years of age or older, pull the pinna upward and backward (Fig. 2).
- Now instill the medication with correct drops, along the side of the ear canal. The dropper should be kept 1–2 cm above the ear canal meatus.
- Keep the child in the same sidelying position for at least 5–7 minutes.
- Keep the cotton ball at the meatus of auditory canal for about 20 minutes to prevent the medication escape outside while the child is in upright position.

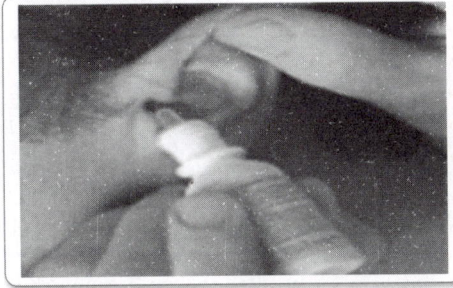
FIG. 2: Instillation of medication into the ear

- Replace the medication and all the articles.
- Do the handwashing properly.
- Assess the child for complications, comfort and discharge from the ear.
- Do the proper recording and reporting of the medications.

NOSE

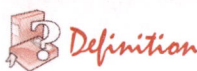 Definition

Administration of medication into the nasal cavity with drop for various therapeutic purposes.

PURPOSES

- To produce local anesthesia for surgical procedures.
- To treat the nasal congestions.
- To treat the sinus infections.
- To treat the allergic reactions.
- To clean the nasal cavity and soften the mucous secreted.

ARTICLES NEEDED

- One pair of gloves.
- Medication with the sterile dropper.
- Child pillow.
- Examination light.
- Face towel.
- Paper bag or kidney tray.

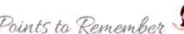 *Points to Remember*

- Identify the patient and his or her name, sex, age, IP number etc.
- Check the physician's order.
- Assess the condition of the child.
- Assess any allergy with medications.
- Nasal drops should be administered 20 minutes before feeding to relieve the congestion.

PROCEDURE

- Do the handwashing properly.
- Explain the procedure to the child if understandable.
- Wear gloves in case of children with nasal drainage.
- Provide proper supine position for access to posterior pharynx, tilt the patient's head backward; for access to ethmoid or sphenoid sinuses, tilt the head back over the edge of bed or we can place small child pillow under the shoulder and tilt the head back.
- Give the support to the child's head with the other hand, and instruct the child to take breath through mouth.
- Place the dropper about 1 cm above the nares and instill the prescribed number of drops towards the midline of ethmoid bone (Fig. 3).

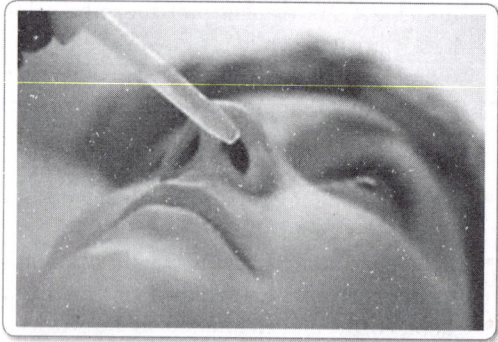

FIG. 3: Instillation of medication into the nose

- Keep the child in supine position for 5 minutes.
- Use a handkerchief or a piece of rag piece to wipe off any medication that has escaped from the anterior nares.
- Provide a sputum mug to spit any medication that has reached the mouth and throat.
- Dispose the soiled supplies and replace all the articles.
- Do the handwashing properly.
- Observe the child for any side effect.
- Do the recording and reporting of the medications.

INTRAMUSCULAR (IM) INJECTION

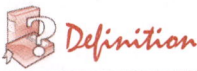 *Definition*

Injection of medications into muscle tissue.

ARTICLES NEEDED

- Injection tray
- Syringe
- Intramuscular 23/24 gauge needle
- Antiseptic solution (spirit)
- Sterile cotton ball jar
- Bottle with antiseptic solution
- Medication prescribed
- Syringe stand and file 20/22 gauge needle to withdraw medication
- Small K-basin
- Medicine card

GENERAL INSTRUCTIONS

- Sites that are commonly used (in children).
- **Thigh:** Anterior aspect of lateral thigh in middle third of vastus lateralis.
  - **Ventrogluteal:** Palpate to locate anterior superior iliac spine and posterior iliac crest; place palm of hand over greater iliac spine and middle finger along crest of posterior by fingers.

IM INJECTION SITES IN CHILDREN

- Vastus lateralis (Fig. 4)
- Ventrogluteal
- Deltoid

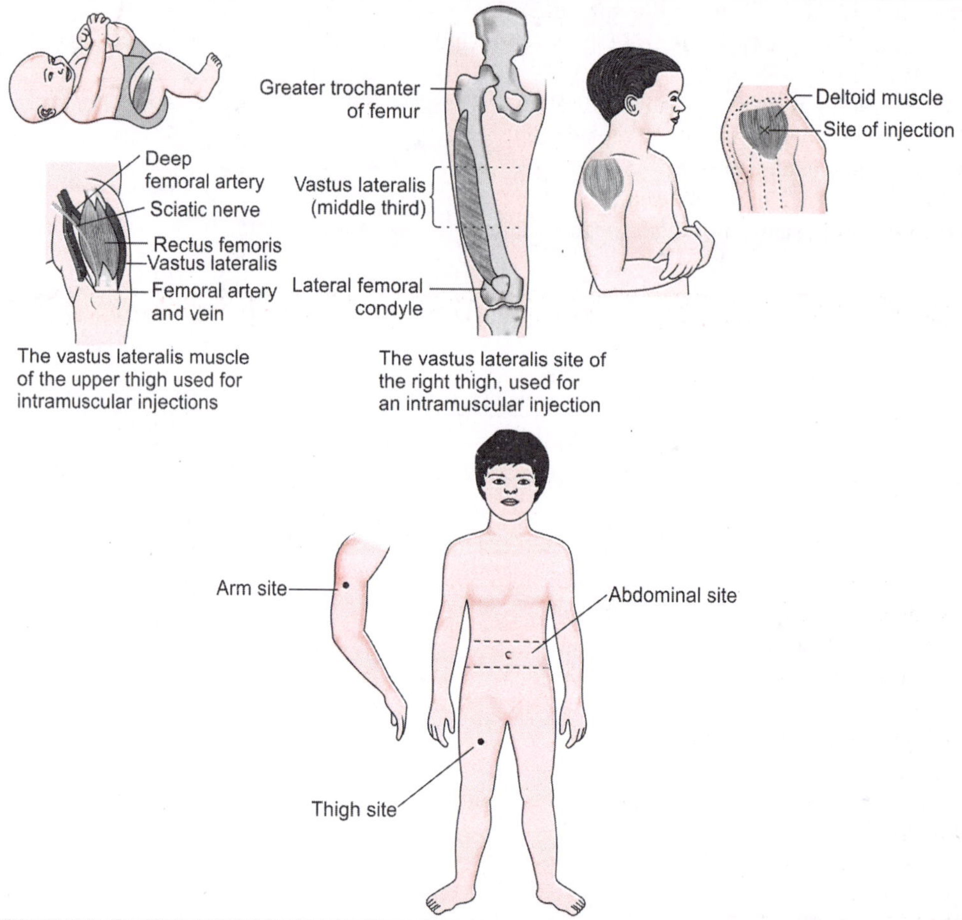

Greater trochanter of femur

Deltoid muscle
Site of injection

Deep femoral artery
Sciatic nerve

Vastus lateralis (middle third)

Rectus femoris
Vastus lateralis
Femoral artery and vein

Lateral femoral condyle

The vastus lateralis muscle of the upper thigh used for intramuscular injections

The vastus lateralis site of the right thigh, used for an intramuscular injection

Arm site

Abdominal site

Thigh site

FIG. 4: Common sites for subcutaneous injections in children

Vastus Lateralis (Fig. 5)

- **Location:** Palpate to find trochanter and knee joints; divide vertical distance between these two landmarks into equal thirds; inject into the middle third.
- **Needle insertion and size:** Insert the needle perpendicular to the knee in infants and young children or perpendicular to the thigh or slightly angled toward the anterior thigh.

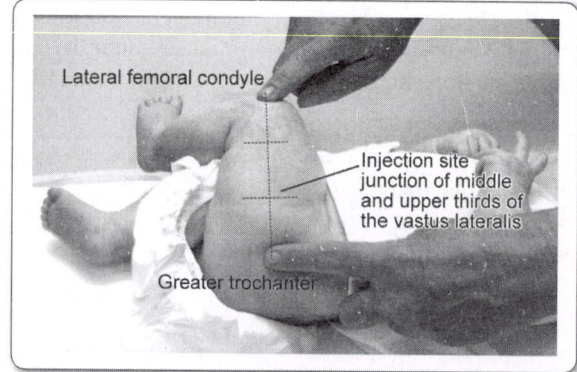

Lateral femoral condyle

Injection site junction of middle and upper thirds of the vastus lateralis

Greater trochanter

FIG. 5: Exact site for injection on vastus lateralis

- **Advantage:**
Large well for developed muscle that can tolerate larger quantities of fluid. (0.5 mL for infant to 2.0 mL for child)
- **Disadvantages:**
  - Thrombosis of femoral artery from injection in mid-thigh area can lead to sciatic nerve damage from long needle injected posteriorly and medially into small extremity.
  - More painful than deltoid or gluteal sites.

Ventrogluteal

- **Location:** Palpate to locate greater trochanter anterior superior iliac tubercles and posterior iliac crest; place palm of hand over greater trochanter, index finger on anterior superior iliac tubercle and middle finger along crest of ileum, posterior as far as possible; inject into canter of 'V' formed by finger.
- **Needle insertion and size:** Insert needle perpendicular to site but angled, slightly toward the iliac crest (20–25 gauge).
- **Advantages:**
  - Free of important nerves and vascular structure.
  - Easily identified by prominent bony landmark.
  - Thinner layer of subcutaneous tissue than in dorsogluteal site, thus less chance of depositing drug subcutaneously rather than intramuscularly. It can accommodate larger quantities of fluid.

Deltoid

- **Location:** Locate acromion process; inject only into upper third of that begins about two finger breadths below acromion.
- **Needle insertion and size:** Insert needle perpendicular to site but angled slightly towards shoulder 22–25 gauge.
- **Advantages:**
  - Faster absorption rates than gluteal sites.
  - Easily accessible with minimal removal of clotting.
  - Less pain and fewer local side effects from vaccines when compared to vastus lateralis.
- **Disadvantages:**
  - Small muscle mass; only limited amount of drug can be injected (0.5–1.0 mL).
  - Small margins of safety with possibility of injury to radial nerve and axillary nerve (not shown, lies under deltoid at head of humerus).

PROCEDURE

- Check, medicine card with patients the chart for name, hospital number, drug to be administered dosages, route of administration and time of administration.
- Prepare medication from ampoule or vial.
- Provide privacy.
- Explain the child or the mother
- Position and expose the appropriate site.
- Determine the correct site for injection.

- Expel the air from the syringe.
- Lean the skin with cotton ball moistened with spirit
- Tighten skin, hold the needle at 90° the angle and insert it swiftly.
- Inject medication slowly and gently.
- Withdraw the needle quickly, place the antiseptic swab just over the injection site.
- Discard both the syringe and needle into the k-basin without disconnecting the needle from syringe.
- Position the child comfortable with itself.
- Record the data, time and name of the drug, dosage and route in nurses, record. Full signature of nurse is mandatory.
- Replace the syringe and needle in disposable unit after completion of procedure according to hospital policy.

SUBCUTANEOUS ADMINISTRATION OF MEDICATION

The drugs which are administered in small amount, such as:
- Heparin and insulin can be introduced by this method.
  - Sites are anterior abdominal wall and inter-scapular areas.

PROCEDURE

- Use small syringe and needle, and draw the medicine.
- Prepare the skin properly.
- Hold the pinch of skin between the thumb and index finger.
- Insert the needle at 45° angle and inject the medicine.
- Discard the waste products.
- Do the recording and reporting of the procedure.

INTRADERMAL INJECTIONS

- Injecting in the right plane is very crucial as it must be restricted to the dermis (just below the epidermis and above the subcutaneous fat).
- These may be needed for giving the Mantoux (tuberculin) test and the BCG vaccine.
- **Site:** The usual site is volar aspect of the left forearm for the mantoux test and skin over the left upper arm for BCG vaccine.
- A 1 mL tuberculin syringe with a 26-gauge needle is used to administer these. The right technique will raise a 0.5 cm wheal of orange peel appearance. It is important to mark the site of mantoux test administration with a pen/marker so that it can be identified for reading after 48–72 hours.

TECHNIQUE OF INTRADERMAL INJECTION

- Use appropriate restraints so that alcohol can denature the proteins in the injected material.
- Do not apply spirit swab to the site.
- After locating the site, stretch the skin between the thumb and the index finger and insert the needle with the bevel facing upwards and needle almost parallel to the skin surface.
- The needle should not be advanced too far or deep under the skin surface and while the medication is being injected, the thin overlying skin becomes raised with an orange peel appearance.

- Remove the needle after injecting the entire amount and do not apply anything on the skin surface.
- Ask the patient to report back after 48–72 hours in case of a mantoux for reading the results.
- For BCG, a small bleb that breaks down to form an ulcer that heals on its own in 6–8 weeks is the normal response.

INTRAVENOUS (IV) INJECTION AND INFUSION (FIG. 6)

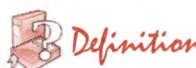 *Definition*

When the medications are introduced through the venous routes, it is known as intravenous injection. These routes are used when medication are introduced in high serum concentration and specifically prescribed by this route only.

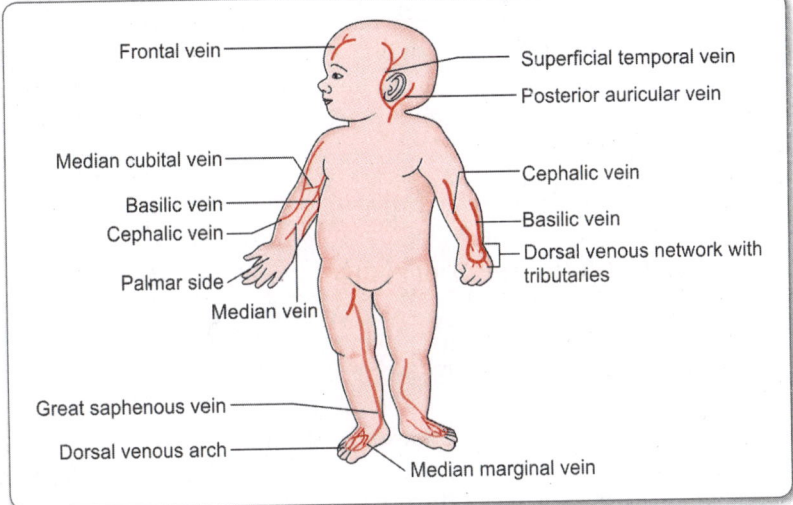

FIG. 6: Intravenous injection

ARTICLES NEEDED

- Adhesive tape
- Syringe disposable (appropriate size)
- Intravenous set (IV set) which includes needle and infusion tube
- Cotton swab (spirit soaked)
- Paper bag or kidney tray for discarding the waste.

Safety Precautions
- Follow the doctor's prescription.
- Follow the aseptic measures.
- Fix the needle with the adhesive tape properly.
- Adjust the proper flow rate as prescribed.
- Provide restraint to the particular extremity if needed.
- Do the proper recording and proper administration of injection.

SITES FOR INTRAVENOUS INFUSION AND INJECTION

There are various routes of IV administration of drugs in children, such as:
- Dorsal arch of hand
- Cephalic vein
- External jugular vein
- Superficial temporal vein
- Frontal vein
- Umbilical vein
- Great saphenous vein
- Dorsal vein (leg), etc.

PROCEDURE

- First locate the vein and clean it with cotton swab.
- Apply the tourniquet between the site chosen and the heart (6–7 cm above the site) to obliterate the venous circulation.
- Ask the child to clench the hands.
- Place the needle in the line with the vein at a 15–45° angle.
- Fix the IV needle with the adhesive tape properly.

PREPARING DIFFERENT STRENGTHS OF IV FLUIDS

Different IV Fluids
- **Dextrose solutions:** 5%, 10%, 25% and 50%.
- **Saline solution:** Normal saline.
- **Dextrose with saline:** Normal saline with 5% dextrose (DNS).
- **Ringer's lactate:** Used for IV rehydration: 130 mEq/L of sodium, 4 mEq/L of potassium, 3 mEq/L of calcium and 28 mEq/L of lactate.
- Isolyte Pt contains 5% dextrose, 30 mEq/L of sodium, 20 mEq/L of potassium.

INDICATIONS

- Neonates with hypoglycaemia, requiring high glucose infusion rates (>4–6 mg/kg/min)
- Electrolyte disturbances: Hyponatraemia, hyperthermia, hyperkalemia
- Post-surgical patients with drains or suctioning from gastrointestinal tract
- Total parental nutrition (TPN) solutions
  Example: Prepare 100 mL of 7.5% dextrose
  Equation: $5(x) + 10(100 - x) = 7.5(100)$
  Answer: 50 mL of 5% dextrose solution and 50 mL of 10% dextrose.

CALCULATIONS OF DRUG DOSAGES AND FLUIDS REQUIREMENTS

The children dosages are calculated on the basis of child's body surface area, age and body weight. There are following formulas used for calculating the dosages for children.

- **According to body surface area:**

  Child dose = $\dfrac{\text{Child's body surface area}}{\text{Adult's body surface area}}$ × Adult dose

- **Young's formula:**

  According to age of child

  Child dose = Age of child in years/Age in years + 12 × adult dose

  Note: This formula is used for children from 1 year to 12 years of age.

- **Clark's formula:**

  According to body weight

  Child dose = Weight of children (in pounds)/150 x adult dose

- **Calculation of body surface area:**
  - Lowe's formula:

    Body surface area (m²) = Weight² (kg) x 0.1
  - Body surface area (m) = 4w + 7/w + 90 where "*w*" is weight in kg

    Fried's formula:

    Child's dose = Age of the child (in months)/150 x adult's dose

    Note: This formula is used for children under one year of age.

FLUID THERAPY

Calculation of Fluid Requirements

Drops Factors

Normal IV set 1 mL = 16 macro drops

Micro volume 1 mL = 60 micro drops

Example:

40 mL/hr = 40 × 16

Macro drops = 40 × 16/60 = 12 drops/min

Micro drops = 40 × 60/60 = 40 drops/min

Formula for Calculation of Daily Fluid Requirements

4:2:1 Method

Body weight	Fluid/Hour	Fluid/Day
0–10 kg	4 mL/kg/h	100/kg/day
11–20 kg	40 mL/kg/h + 2 mL/h	1000 mL + 50 mL/kg for each kg
Above 20 kg	60 mL/kg/h + 1 mL/kg/h	1500 mL + 20 mL for each kg

NOTES: 4 mL/kg/h for first 10 kg; adding first 10 kg 1000 mL/day + (50 mL/each kg/day); adding 2 mL/kg/h for second 10 kg; adding first 20 kg 1500 mL/day + (20 mL/each kg/day) and adding 1 mL/kg/h for each kg over 20 kg

Calculating the Flow Rate

Intravenous fluid (Drops) calculation formula:

= Total volume of fluid (mL) × 15 drops/Total hours × 60

OR

Drop per minute = Total volume/Time in minutes × drop factor

Fluid Replacement Formula

Fluid replacement formula in burn cases is dependent on the total body surface area (TBSA) burnt and bodyweight of the child. There are various formulas used for fluid replacement, among them parkland formula is commonly used.

Parkland Formula

For First 24 Hours

Total amount of fluid requirement = 4 mL of ringer's lactate × weight in kg × percentage of TBSA burnt.
   One half of the fluid should be given in first 8 hours, start from the time of accident.
   Remaining half of the fluid should be given in the next 16 hours.

For Next 24 Hours

Total amount of fluid requirement = 2 mL of ringer's lactate (RL) per kg per % of burns.
   This formula is used when the burn is 15–20% of total body surface area (TBSA).

Preparing the Solution by Using a Formula

In case of diluted medicines, the following formula will be helpful to find out the strength of the solution.
   Amount of stock solution required (A) = Desired strength (d)/Strength of what we have in stock (H) × Quantity required (Q)

Neonatal Fluid Requirements

Total fluids administered are increased on a daily basis by 10–15 mL/kg/day increments, up to a maximum of 150 mL/kg/day by the end of first week of life. Sodium and potassium are added in intravenous fluids from day 3 of life. In case of prematurity, IUGR and for those who are born to diabetic mothers, it may be necessary to add calcium gluconate (10% solution: 8 mL/kg/day) to initial intravenous fluids to prevent hypocalcemia (Table 1).

TABLE 1: Daily fluid requirements in the first week of life (mL/kg)

Age in days	<1000 g	1000–1500 g	>1500 g
1	80	80	60
2	100	95	75
3	120	110	90
4	130	120	105
5	140	130	120
6	150	140	135
7	160	150	150

FLUIDS IN SPECIAL SITUATIONS

- **In case of fever:** 12.5% extra fluid should be added for every degree centigrade rise in temperature above 38°C.
- **Neonates under warmer/phototherapy:** 20 mL/kg/day needs to be added to the maintenance fluid requirements.

- **Shock:** 20 mL/kg normal saline or ringer's lactate, and it will be repeated every 10–20 minutes based on ongoing assessment.
- **Renal failure:** Insensible losses 300–400 mL/m² of body surface area are replaced volume for every 6 hours by 10% dextrose, while urine output is replaced by half NS (N/2 saline)
- **Chemotherapy:** 3 L/m² body surface area, with sodium bicarbonate.

Dehydration (Tables 2 and 3)

TABLE 2: Dehydration assessment tool

Signs	A	B	C	D
Step 1				Shock
Look at general conditions	Well alert	Irritable and restless	Floppy, lethargic or unconscious	Unconscious not able to drink
Eyes	Eyes are normal	Sunken eyes	Sunken eyes	
Thirst	Not thirsty and drinks normally	Thirsty and drinks eagerly	Drinks poorly or not able to drink	
Step 2				
Feel				
Pinch the skin	Goes back immediately	Goes back slowly	Goes back very slowly more than 2 seconds	As in C plus capillary refill more than 3 seconds, cold hands
Step 3				
Decide	No signs of dehydration	Two or more signs means	Two or more signs means	Shock
Degree of dehydration		Some dehydration	Severe dehydration	
Step 4				
Treat	Use treatment plan A	Use treatment plan B	Use treatment plan C urgently	Treat shock very urgently

TABLE 3: Signs in various degrees of dehydration

Signs	Mild	Moderate	Severe
Severe weight loss	Up to 5%	6–10%	More than 10%
Appearance	Active, alert	Irritable, alert, thirsty	Lethargic, looks sick
Capillary filling (compared to your own)	Normal	Slightly delayed	Delayed
Pulse	Normal	Fast, low volume	Very fast, thread
Respiration	Normal	Fast	Fast and deep
Blood pressure	Normal	Normal or low orthostatic hypotension	Very low
Mucous membranes	Moist	Dry	Parched
Tears	Present	Less than expected	Absent

Contd...

Signs	Mild	Moderate	Severe
Eyes	Normal	Normal	Sunken
Pinched skin	Springs back	Tents briefly	Prolonged tenting
Fontanel (infant sitting)	Normal	Sunken slightly	Sunken significantly
Urine flow	Normal	Reduced	Severely reduced

Management of Dehydration

Immediate aim of therapy is to administer fluids and electrolytes lost which is completed in 6–8 hours.

Approximate amount of fluid needed is 50, 100 and 150 mL/kg for mild, moderate and severe dehydration, respectively, in infants. In young children, three/fourth and in older children two/third of this is given.

TABLE 4: Composition of the various types of correction fluids

Dehydration	N saline	5% glucose	7.5% NaHCO$_3$	15% KCL
Hypotonic	600	400	30	10
Isotonic	400	600	30	10
Hypertonic	200	800	30	10

Fluid should be given more rapidly during the first 1–2 hours at the rate of 20 mL/kg/h, and thereafter adjusted to deliver the rest of the fluids.

Prevention of dehydration is corrected by fluid management.

The amount of ORS required is:

- <2 years 50–100 mL/loose motion
- 2–10 years 100–200 mL/loose motion
- >10 years as much as wanted

Prevention of Some Dehydration

Give 75 mL/kg ORS in the first 4 hours; if the child wants more than calculate and give ORS.

Prevention of Severe Dehydration

- <1 year: 30 mL/kg in the first hour
  - 70 mL/kg in the next 5 hours
  - >1-year-old: 30 mL/kg in first 30 minutes and rest in the next 2.5 hours

8

Administrations of Medication to Children

● *Oral Medication*

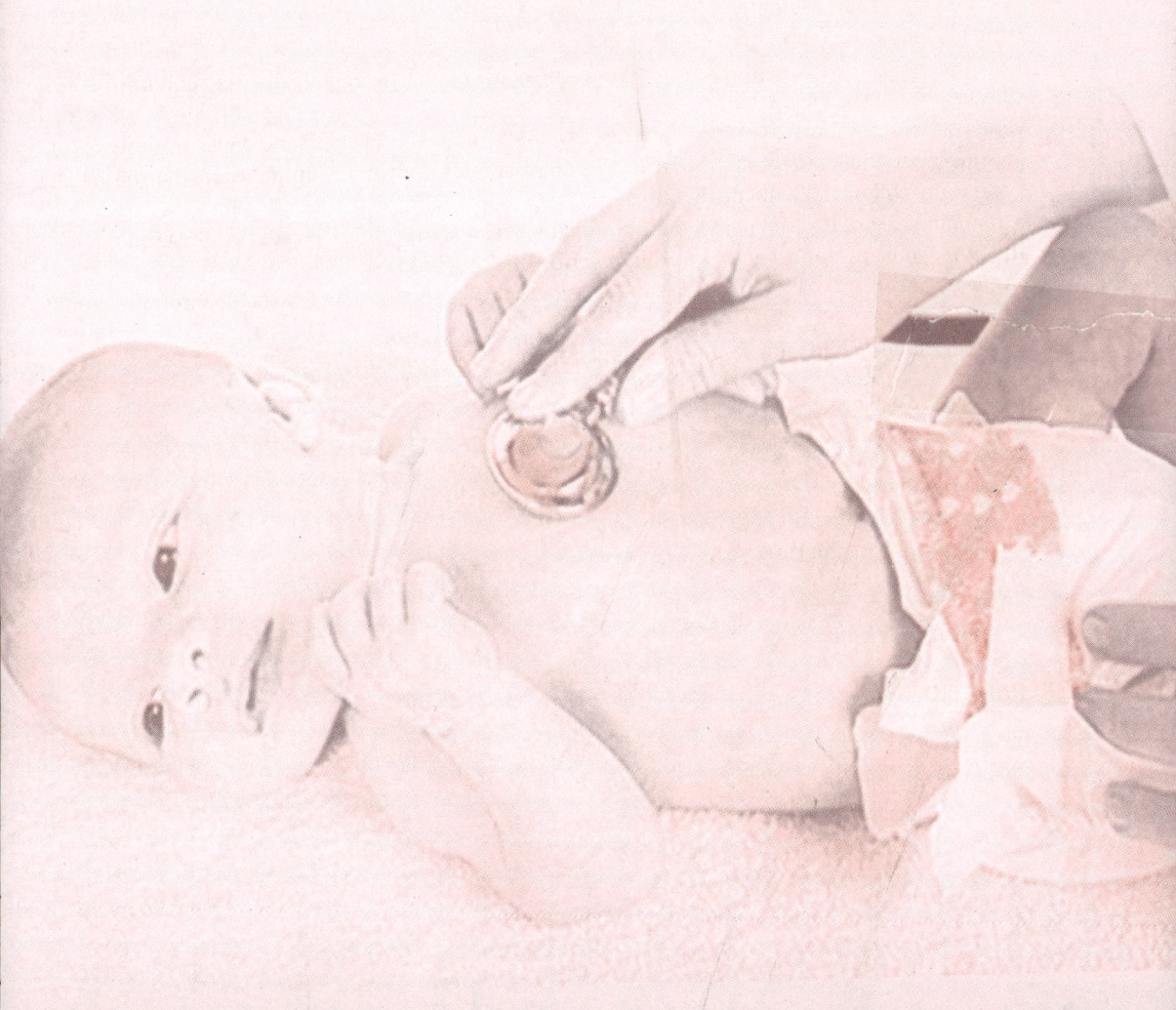

LEARNING OBJECTIVES

On completion of this chapter, the pediatric nurse will be able to perform the following activities:
- Explain principles of administration of oral medication of children
- Preparation of medications
- Develop skills in administration of oral medication.

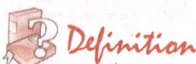 *Definition*

The oral route administration is preferred for administering medications to children because of the ease of administration. Most of the medications are dissolved or suspended in liquid preparations.

GENERAL GUIDELINES

- The responsibility of giving medications to children is a serious one.
- Half of all medications in the market today do not have a documented safe use in children.
- Children are smaller than adults and medication dosage must be adjusted.
- Children react more violently.
- Drug reactions are not predictable.
- The impact on growth and development must be considered when giving drugs to children.
- Double checking is always best.
- Pediatric drug therapy should be guided by the child's age, weight and level of growth and development. The nurse's approach to the child should convey the impression that he or she expects the child to take the medication.
- Explanation regarding the medications should be based on the child's level of understanding.
- The nurse must be honest with the child regarding the procedure.
- It may be necessary to mix distasteful medication or crushed tablets with a small amount of honey and gelatin.
- Never threaten a child with an injection if he/she refuses an oral medication.

THINGS TO TAKE CARE

- Infant/child cries and refuses to take medication or spits it out.
- Do not use in case of vomiting, malabsorption or refusal by the child.
- Kids <5 years find it difficult to swallow tablets.
- Use suspension or chewable forms.
- Divide only scored tablets.
- Empty capsules in a jelly.
- Do not call medication 'candy'.

PREPARATION

- The devices available to measure medicines are not always sufficiently accurate for measuring the small amounts needed in pediatric nursing practice.

- Molded plastic caps offer reasonable accuracy in measuring moderate doses of liquids; paper cups, on the other hand, are likely to have irregularly shaped or crumpled bottoms and retain considerable amounts of thick medication.
- Measures less than 1 teaspoon are impossible to determine accurately with a medicine cup.
- The teaspoon is an inaccurate measuring device and is subject to error.
- Teaspoons vary greatly in capacity, different persons using the same spoon will pour different amounts.
- Therefore, measures a drug ordered in teaspoon in milliliters; the established standard is 5 mL/tsp.
- Household measuring spoons can also be used when other devices are not available.
- Another unreliable device for measuring liquids is the dropper, which varies, to a greater extent, with the teaspoon or measuring cup.
- It is best to place the dropper or syringe along the side of the infant's tongue and administer the liquid slowly in small amounts, waiting for the child to swallow between deposits.

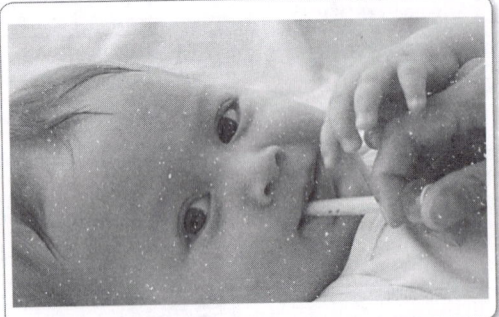

FIG. 1. Using a dropper as a method for oral administration

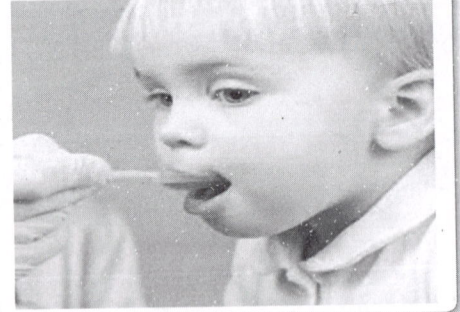

FIG. 2: Using spoon as a mode for oral administrations

- Medicine cups can be used effectively for older infants who are able to drink from a cup.
- Allowing the infant to suck the medication that has been placed in an empty nipple or inserting the syringe or dropper into the side of the mouth, parallel to the nipple.
- Mix with small amount of juice or fruit, give in syringe or allow the child to hold the medicine cup and drink it at his/her own pace if he/she is big enough.
- Parent can also give the medication if the nurse is present in the room.
- **Older child:** Tell the child to drink juice after distasteful medication. Older children can suck the medication from a syringe, pinch their nose, or drink through a straw to decrease the input of smell, which adds to the unpleasantness of oral medication.

Nursing alert: For liquid medications, an oral syringe or medication cup should be used to ensure accurate dosage measurement. Use of a household teaspoon or tablespoon may result in dosage error because these are inaccurate measures.

- **Documentation:**
  - Date, time, name of the drug, dose, route and signature and side effects
  - Report: Report to ward in charge.

PROCEDURE

Step/task
Wash hands with soap and water
Take a clean spoon and place half tablet for children ages 2 months up to 6 months and 1 tablet for a child of 6 months up to 5 years
Pour mother's breast milk or clean water in the spoon
Allows the tablet to disperse (30 seconds to 1 minute). Check that the tablet is completely dissolved
Ask the mother to give the prepared medicine to the baby in her presence. If some portion of the medicine is left in the spoon, put little breast milk or water and give it to the child

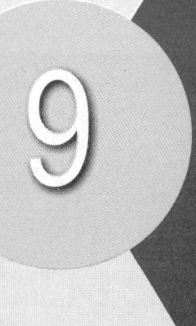

Specimen Collection

- Urine Specimen
- Stool Specimen
- Sputum Specimen
- Blood Specimen

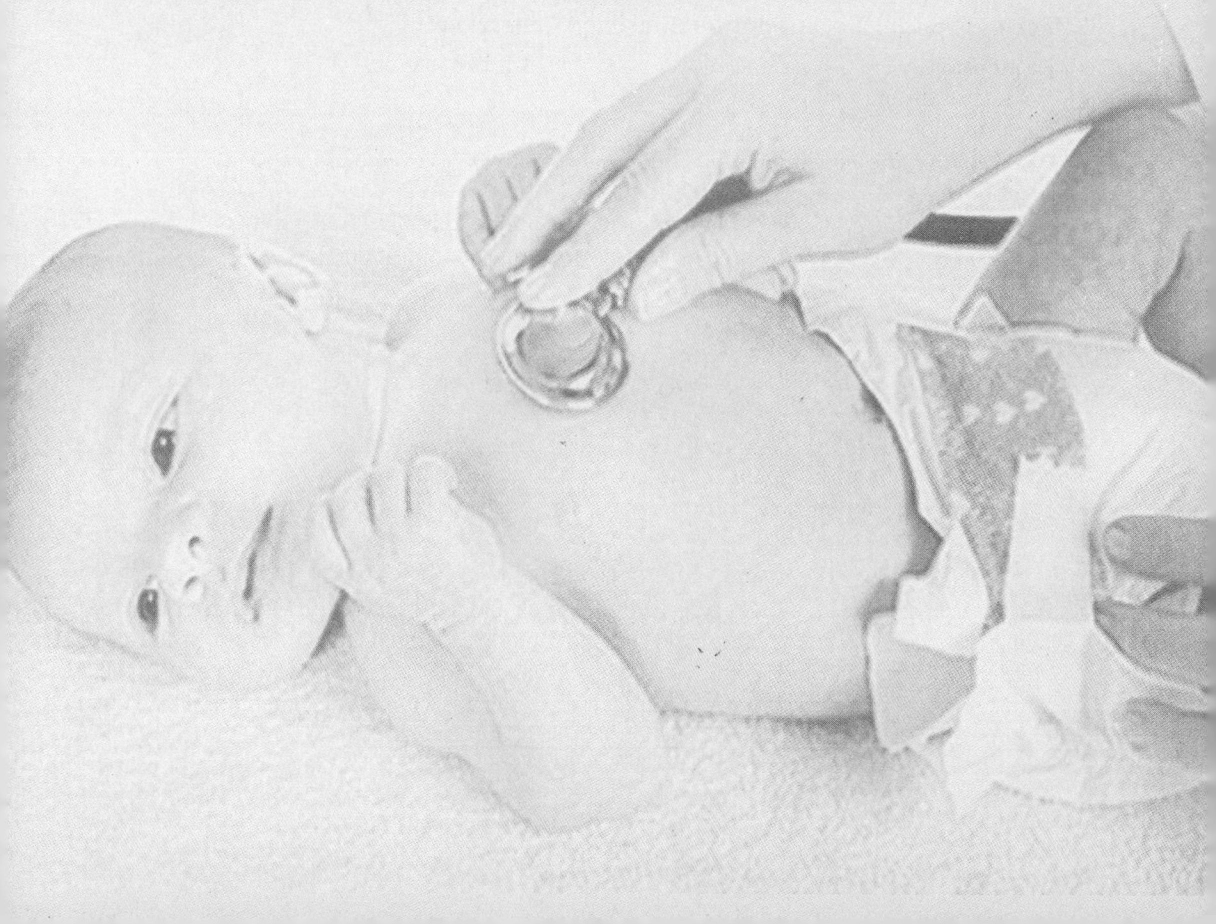

LEARNING OBJECTIVES

On the completion of this chapter, the pediatric nurse will be able to perform the following activities:
- Explain purposes and methods of collection of different specimens
- Develop skills in these procedures
- Inculcate the same in their practical field.

SPECIMEN COLLECTION

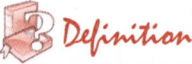 Definition

Specimen may be defined as a small quantity of a substance or object which shows the total qualitative characteristics. The accuracy and reliability of findings depend upon the correct method of collection, transportation of the specimen to the laboratory and recording of reports. Inaccurate results may mislead the physician in the diagnosis and treatment of the patient.

Purposes of Specimen Collection

- To confirm the diagnosis.
- To provide the appropriate treatment based on results.
- To detect the effectiveness of treatment plan and any abnormalities.

Safety and Special Precautions for Specimen Collection

- Equipment used for specimen collection should be clean or sterile.
- Do not use any antiseptics in specimen.
- Check the physician order properly.
- When culture specimen is required, the container should be covered properly with lid. Do not open it unnecessarily.
- Specimen should always be fresh for laboratory examination.
- Wherever necessary, add the preservatives to prevent decomposition.
- Label the specimen as early as possible.
- Send the specimen with the proper requisition. Form should be duly filled in and signed by authority.
- Do not misplace the specimen.
- Use proper size containers according to nature of specimens and no cracks should be there in the container.
- Always use a wide mouth container to prevent spilling.
- Do not contaminate the containers outside with the specimen.
- Do the proper recording and reporting.

Collection of Specimen

- **Patient preparation:** Explain the procedure to the child if the child is able to understand. In case of urine specimen if the child is male, clean the buttocks of the child with cotton swab soaked in sterile water. Wash the groin, scrotum and penis with the soap and clean water. Then, dry the areas with sterile dry cotton swab. The penis and urethral meatus should be cleaned properly with moist cotton balls. Dry the area with sterile cotton balls and do not touch the penis unnecessarily after cleaning. If the child is female, place the child in a semirecumbent position. Clean the buttocks, external genitalia with soap and water. Clean the surrounding area to prevent contamination. Clean the labia minora and majora with sterile cotton balls soaked in sterile water. Cleaning should be done by following the stroke from above to downwards. Use one cotton swab with one stroke.

- **Equipment preparation:** Specimens should be collected in properly clean or sterile container. Disposable cups are used to collect the stool or sputum specimens. For fluid collection, use sterile tubes. For smears, use sterile slides. For children (neonates), use a sterile urine bag. Specimen containers should have a wide mouth. Do not use any antiseptic solution in the specimen. Do not touch the mouth of the specimen container.

URINE SPECIMEN

It involves collection of urine for the therapeutic purposes and sending it to the laboratory for test (Fig. 1).

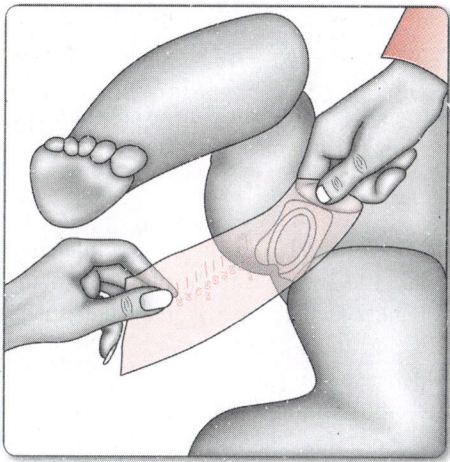

FIG. 1: Urine collection

Purposes

- To find out the presence of abnormalities like red blood cells (haematuria, white blood cells etc.)
- To check the sugar, albumin and pH
- To check the specific gravity
- To detect the cause of urinary tract infections
- To finalise the diagnosis and recommendation of treatment

Articles Needed

- Sterile cotton swab in a bowl soaked with sterile water, and one bowl with dry cotton balls for cleaning the area
- Water with soap
- Urinal or bedpan
- Clean, sterile or disposable containers with wide neck and mouth
- Urine bag (disposable)
- Kidney tray or paper bag for discarding the waste products.

Types of Specimen

- **Mid-stream urine specimen:** In mid-stream of urine, the first stream of urine is flushed out and removes the organisms and mucus is usually present at the meatus. By this process, accurate result can be obtained. Explain the procedure to the child. The child should be encouraged to pass the urine in the bedpan and after the some amount of urine has been voided, collect the mid-stream of urine in a sterile specimen bottle as needed. Clean the outer surface of the bottle with a sterile swab and label it properly.
- **Single urine specimen:** Single urine specimen includes amount of urine voided at a time. In this, usually morning urine specimens are collected. For this about 100–150 mL of urine will be adequate for the laboratory tests. In this method, the child passes urine directly into the specimen bottle after the cleaning of genitalia. Cover the container as early as possible and label it properly.
- **24-hour urine specimen:** It includes the collection of urine voided in 24 hours. It starts at 6 am and urine voided in the whole day is collected in a specimen bottle or in a disposable urine bag (uro-bag) till next morning 6 am. In this method, we should add the preservatives to the urine to prevent the decomposition and multiplication of bacteria or organisms.
- **Routine urine specimen by bag:** Today pediatric urine collection bags are available in the market. This method is used for the neonates, infants and those who can not control the bladder.

Procedure

- The nurse should wash the hands properly and clean the genitalia of the child properly.
- Wash the hands again and place the urine bag to the perineum of the female child.
- The opening of the urine bag should be fitted properly around the genitalia and fixed with adhesive tapes.
- Keep the child in semi-Fowler position.
- Urine bag for the boys should be used properly.
- In this process the penis and scrotum should be inserted into the opening of the bag.
- If needed, provide restraint to the child.
- Nursing personnel should observe properly to prevent the leaking of urine from the bag. After voiding the urine, the urine bag should be removed and the specimen should be sent to the laboratory for completing the desired tests.

Urine Specimen by Catheter

It is available in different sizes. Choose the catheter according to age and insert it properly and gently. The specimen is directly collected into the sterile container and sent to the laboratory.

Complications

This method in children can cause:
- Injury to the genital organs, especially urethra
- Risk of infections is more
- It is discomforting to the child.

STOOL SPECIMEN

It is a collection of small amount of stool for the therapeutic and diagnostic purposes.

Purposes

- To detect the organisms such as *Shigella, Salmonella*, etc.
- To find out the abnormal stool characteristics such as color, odor, consistency and form and composition etc.

Articles Needed

- Specimen container with a wide mouth
- Sterile stick or wooden spatula
- Bedpans
- Pair of gloves
- Disposable tissue paper
- Waste bin for discarding the waste.

Procedure

- Explain the procedure to the patient regarding the defecation of stool in bedpan.
- Provide a clean sterile specimen container to the patient with spatula, if he/she is able to do.
- Advise the patient how to take the specimen with spatula and transfer it into the specimen container. If the child is not able to perform, it should be completed by the caregiver or a trained person.
- After collection of specimen in the container, label it properly and send it to the laboratory for the desired test.
- Spatula should be wrapped in tissue paper and discarded in waste bin.
- Wash and dry the hands.
- Record and report the observations.

SPUTUM SPECIMEN

Sputum specimen is collected from the coughed out sputum to detect the respiratory pathogens for therapeutic purposes.

Articles Needed

- A test tube/sterile specimen container
- Sputum cup
- Cotton applicator
- Tissue paper to clean the mouth
- Pair of gloves
- Recording and reporting articles.

Procedure

- Identify the patient and check the physician's order.
- Explain the procedure to the patient.
- Make the patient sit comfortably.
- Keep the sterile container and tissue paper near the bedside of the patient.
- Advise the patient take deep breath and cough out deeply from the lungs.

- Open the lid of the container and expectorate inside the container and close it immediately.
- When a specimen is from young child, we can use a cotton applicator and a test tube. When sputum is coughed up, wipe off the sputum with cotton applicator and let is drop into the clean test tube. Close the test tube with a cotton plug.
- Label the container/test tube and send it to the laboratory for the examination.
- Clean the mouth with tissue paper.
- Clean the articles and replace them.
- Wash the hands properly.

BLOOD SPECIMEN

It includes collecting the small amount of blood in sterile containers/test tubes for various therapeutic purposes.

Purposes

- To measure the blood Hb level, blood urea, blood glucose, random blood sugar level, bilirubin level, count of WBC, RBC, etc.
- To detect malarial parasites
- To check HIV, hepatitis etc.
- To find out the abnormal composition of blood
- To aid in confirmation of diagnosis
- To check the effectiveness of treatment
- To help in the planning of treatment.

Articles Needed

- Specimen container—bottle or test tube
- Tourniquet
- Slides (if blood smear is needed)
- 5 mL syringes
- Sterile (disposable) needle
- Spirit-soaked cotton swab in a container
- Pair of gloves
- Adhesive tapes
- Kidney tray or paper bag for waste discard
- Recording and reporting articles

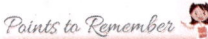 *Points to Remember*

- Explain the procedure to the patient and reassure about the pain and blood sample.
- Provide him or her a comfortable position for sitting or supine position; young and infant children cannot understand the procedure, so provide them mummy restraint.
- Wash the hands and wear the gloves.

Preferred Sites for Venipuncture

In infant's femoral vein, antecubital fossa should be punctured; other suitable routes are wrist, dorsum (back) of the hand and top area of foot.

Procedure

- Extend the arm and clench the fist.
- Tourniquet should be applied 5–15 cm above the selected sites to obstruct the blood flow from the vein.
- Prepare the skin by cleaning it with spirit or alcohol swab in circular motion from center to periphery.
- Remove the cap of needle and connect it with syringe. Insert the needle smoothly into the vein.
- If the needle is inserted in the vein properly, blood comes out speedily in the syringe. Now collect the specimen in the syringe by pulling the plunger back slowly.
- When specimen is collected completely, open the tourniquet and fist.
- At the site of venipuncture, apply cotton swab and fix with adhesive tape or apply the pressure over the site with finger for 3–5 minutes, to prevent the leakage of blood.
- Transfer the blood specimen into the container. Label it and send it early to the lab for the desired test.

Taking Blood Smear

- Clean the child's tip of finger with spirit, turn the face of the child to one side and press the finger tip and give a gentle prick with sterile needle. Take the blood on the slide and make smear on slides. A cotton swab should be applied on the fingertip at the site of pin prick and adhesive tape or pressure should be applied to stop the bleeding.
- In infants, peripheral capillary blood samples can be obtained from the earlobe stab, tip of fingers and heel stick.
- All the articles should be cleaned and waste products should be discarded.
- Replace all the articles.
- Record and report the results properly.

Femoral Puncture

Procedure

- Infant lies supine on the edge of the table with legs firmly pulled down in abdomen.
- Legs are held by an assistant above the patient and the arms of the infant are held down by the assistant's arm and elbows.
- The entire inguinal area is cleaned aseptically.
- Femoral artery is palpated below the inguinal ligament and skin punctured medial to it, 3–4 cm below inguinal ligament and needle inserted to a depth of 0.5–0.75 cm.
- Apply constant suction, and needle is slowly withdrawn until blood enters the syringe. If a continuous flow is not obtained, the needle is pushed a little deeper and then withdrawn as before.
- Firm pressure is applied for several minutes after withdrawal of the needle to avoid haematoma formation.

External Jugular Puncture

Infant is immobilized by mummifying and turned to one side.

Procedure

- The area is cleaned aseptically.
- The child is provoked to cry, which makes the vein prominent.

- Alternatively, it is made prominent by pressing at the lower end.
- Vein is entered with a butterfly needle attached to a syringe.
- Pressure is applied at the puncture site and the child held upright.

Internal Jugular Puncture

Procedure

- The child is mummified, neck extended and turned slightly to one side to make the opposite sternomastoid muscle prominent.
- The area is cleaned aseptically.
- A needle is inserted along the posterior border of the sternomastoid muscle, midway between the tip of mastoid process and the sternoclavicular joint.
- The needle is advanced in the direction of suprasternal notch (tip of the left index finger placed at the notch helps as a guide) under constant suction, until the blood enters the syringe.
- In case no blood comes out, the needle is withdrawn under suction.

Scalp Vein Puncture

- Scalp is shaved and cleaned aseptically.
- A tourniquet may be tied to make the veins prominent.
- Rubbing alcohol also helps.
- Vein is punctured with a butterfly needle (no. 21 or 23).
- Skin is pierced 0.5 cm distal and slightly to one side of venipuncture site.

Arterial Blood

- Femoral, brachial, radial arteries may be used.
- Skin is cleaned aseptically and artery located by palpation.
- As the needle enters arterial lumen, blood flows out into the syringe automatically.
- Firm pressure must be maintained over the puncture site for 3–5 min. after needle withdrawal.

Complications

- Haematoma
- Septic arthritis and femoral artery spasm
- Sudden blanching of the limb and cessation of femoral artery pulsation indicate artery spasm: immediate infiltration of the surrounding area with lignocaine is indicated.

NOTE: All the specimens should be properly labeled with the following details.

Box 1

Name of the patient ....
Age of patient ....
Bed No. .... Ward No..
OPD/IPD No...
Name of specimen ....
Name of the test done...
Date of collection of specimen ....
Signature of nurse/authority...

10

Care of Baby in an Incubator

- Purposes
- Parts of an Incubator
- Steps of Procedure

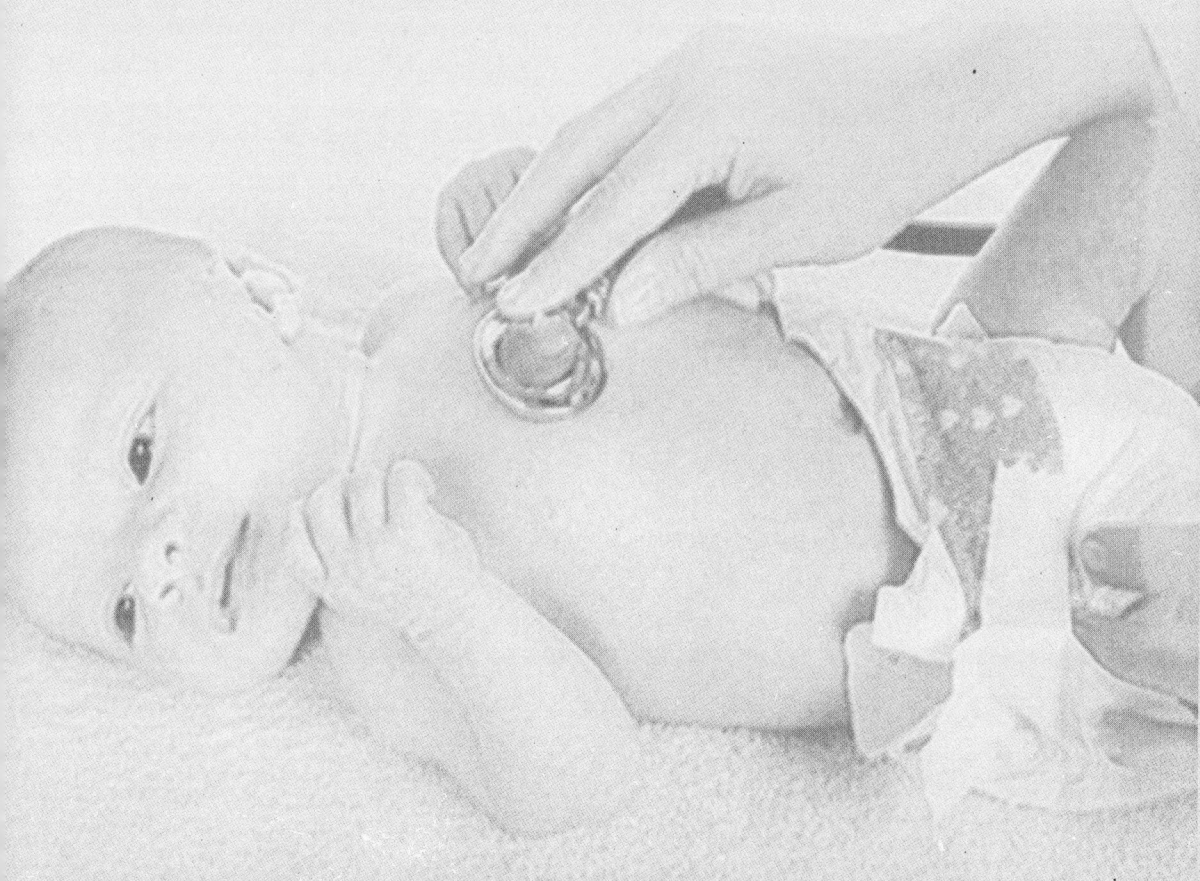

LEARNING OBJECTIVES

On the completion of this chapter, the pediatric nurse will be able to perform the following activities:
- Explain the purposes and different types of equipment
- Develop skills in care of the children under various procedures
- Inculcate these skills in their practical field

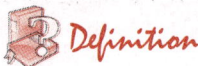 *Definition*

Incubator is an electronic based device which is used to maintain the condition of high-risk, preterm babies.

PURPOSES

- To maintain the body temperature in case of premature babies
- To provide the oxygen to the baby
- To maintain humidity around the baby
- To protect the baby from the infections
- To observe the baby.

PARTS OF AN INCUBATOR

Incubator consists of the following parts:
- Deck
- A mattress which is enclosed by clear plastic canopy
- Air intake pipe
- Thermostat
- Oxygen inlet
- Two arm ports
- **Hood:** It is rectangular in shape. Hood has a large door for placing or removing the baby from the incubator. It has four elbow-operated parts for doing the small procedures. It has inlet for IV tubes, endotracheal tubes and probes. When there is need of cleaning, canopy can be lifted.
- **Control panel:** It aims to electronically control the temperature.
- **Lower unit:** This unit contains the control box, touch sensor, front panel, humidifier, air ducts and air filters. The front panel displays patient body temperature, air temperature, control temperature, alarm mute or on, power off or on etc.
- **Cabinet:** Cabinet gives support to the hood, canopy and lower unit. Cabinet has a main switch, fuse and power cord connector. Some cabinets have drawers two or three for storage.
- **Humidity maintenance:** In the incubator, air is circulated by the blower. Fresh air enters through the air filters which are located at the end of the incubator canopy and passed over the heater and humidifier. The temperature inside the incubator is maintained by the sensor placed on the hood, which helps heated air flow to the surrounding of the infant.

STEPS OF PROCEDURE (FIG. 1)

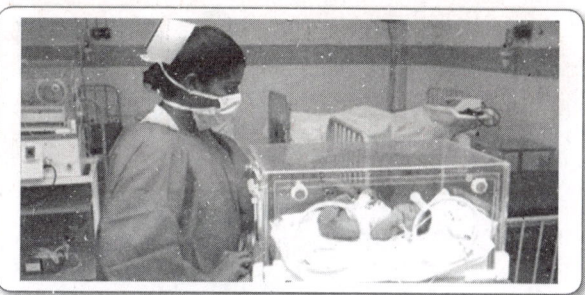

FIG. 1: Care of the baby in an incubator

- Identify the baby and check physician's order.
- Procedure or care can be explained to the parents.
- Clean the incubator with disinfecting solutions before placing the baby; canopy should also be cleaned.
- Switch on the incubator and adjust the temperature by the front control panel. Temperature should be at about 36°C.
- The oxygen inlet should be connected to the oxygen source.
- Warm the incubator for at least 15–20 minutes before placing the baby.
- Keep the bay in the incubator properly and undress the baby except the diapers, and change the diaper regularly as the need arises.
- Temperature of the baby and incubator should be checked every hour, until the temperature of baby is stabilized.
- Report to doctor if the baby is not maintaining normal temperature for two consecutive readings
- Humidifier water should be changed everyday.
- Provide the care to the baby by introducing the hand through the arm ports only.
- Do not open the incubator unnecessarily; open at the time of need only.
- Allow the visiting of parents for their satisfaction and increase mother–child bond as policy.
- Wash hands before touching the infant and after giving the care.
- Place the incubator at a proper, safe place. Do not place it near the doors.
- Avoid tap to incubator to prevent disturbance to the baby.
- The infants should be warmly wrapped in a blanket after taking out from an incubator.
- The power plug of incubator should not have any sparking to avoid any fire hazards.
- Maintain continuous observation on the baby during incubator care.
- Documents
  - Time and temperature of the baby
  - Set temperature of the incubator

11

Care of Baby in Radiant Warmer

- ➲ Purposes
- ➲ Parts of Radiant Warmer
- ➲ Steps of Procedure
- ➲ Cautions

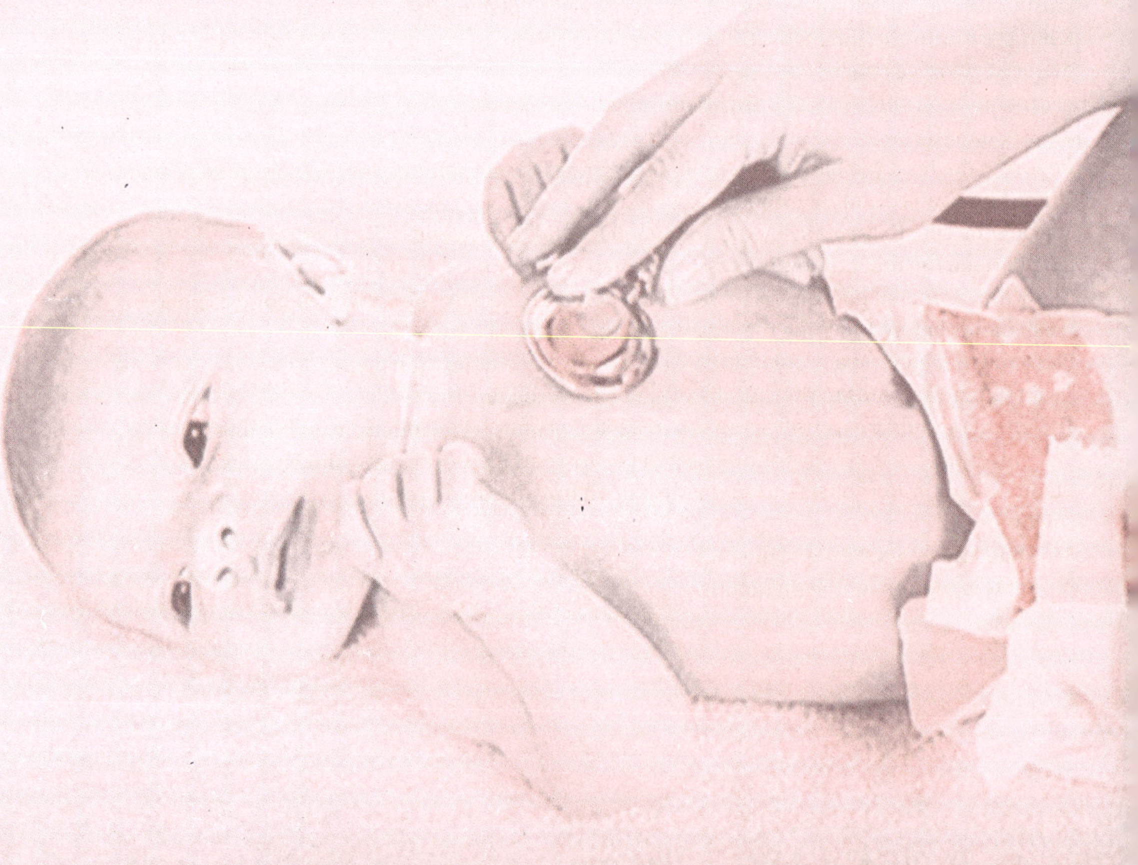

LEARNING OBJECTIVES

On the completion of this chapter, the pediatric nurse will be able to perform the following activity:
- Provide care to the baby in radiant warmer

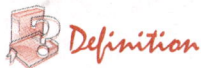 *Definition*

Radiant warmer (Fig. 1) is an electronically based device which is used to maintain the body temperature.

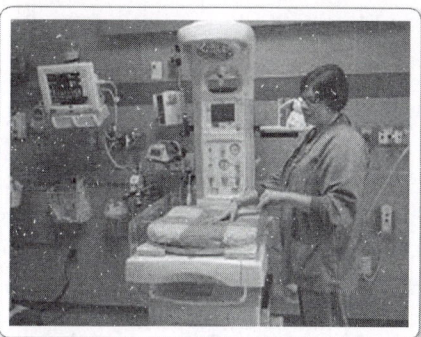

FIG. 1: Radiant warmer

PURPOSES

- To maintain the baby temperature just after the birth.
- To observe the child under proper light source.
- To suction or resuscitate the baby in case of any obstruction or any cyanotic episodes.
- To introduce the medication for long duration, e.g. IV (intravenous) administration.

PARTS OF RADIANT WARMER

- Mattress as platform to place the baby.
- Side rails to prevent the baby from falling.
- Light source to examine the baby.
- Control panel to maintain the temperature, of skin, set the alarm and indicator of power on/off.
- IV stand.
- Side tray for keeping the medications, feeding materials and oxygen hood.
- Warmer filaments or rods to keep the baby warm.

Cautions

- Infant should not be left unattended when the radiant warmer is being used in manual mode.
- Measures to maintain desired fluid balance should be considered since open radiant warming causes insensible water loss.
- No naked flame should be there
- No smoking should be done

STEPS OF PROCEDURE

CAUTIONS

- Switch on the machine at least 20 minutes prior to the expected time of delivery/arrival of the low birth weight or sick babies
- Identify in the temperature panel that the readings are set as skin temperature and the air temperature
- Identify servo and manual mode switches
- Set the warmer in manual mode
- Adjust the heat output to:
  - High: If baby's temperature is below 36°C
  - Medium: If baby's temperature is between 36°C and 36.5°C
  - Low: If baby's temperature is between 36.5°C and 37.5°C
- Switch to servo control mode setting once the temperature of the baby is between 36.5°C and 37.4°C
- Place the baby on the bassinet. Identify the correct site (*right hypochondrium in supine position*) and connect skin probe to the baby's abdomen with sticking tape
- Set alarm (Set the desired temperature of baby to be maintained between 36.5°C and 37.4°C)
- Ensure that the baby's head is covered with a cap and feet are secured in socks; the baby is clothed or covered unless it is necessary for the baby to be naked or partially undressed for observation or for a procedure
- Respond to alarm immediately and identify the fault and rectify it
- Check the sensor probe regularly so as to ensure that it is in place

12

Care of Baby in Phototherapy

- ➲ Purpose
- ➲ Parts of Phototherapy Unit
- ➲ Types
- ➲ Articles Needed
- ➲ Care to the Baby

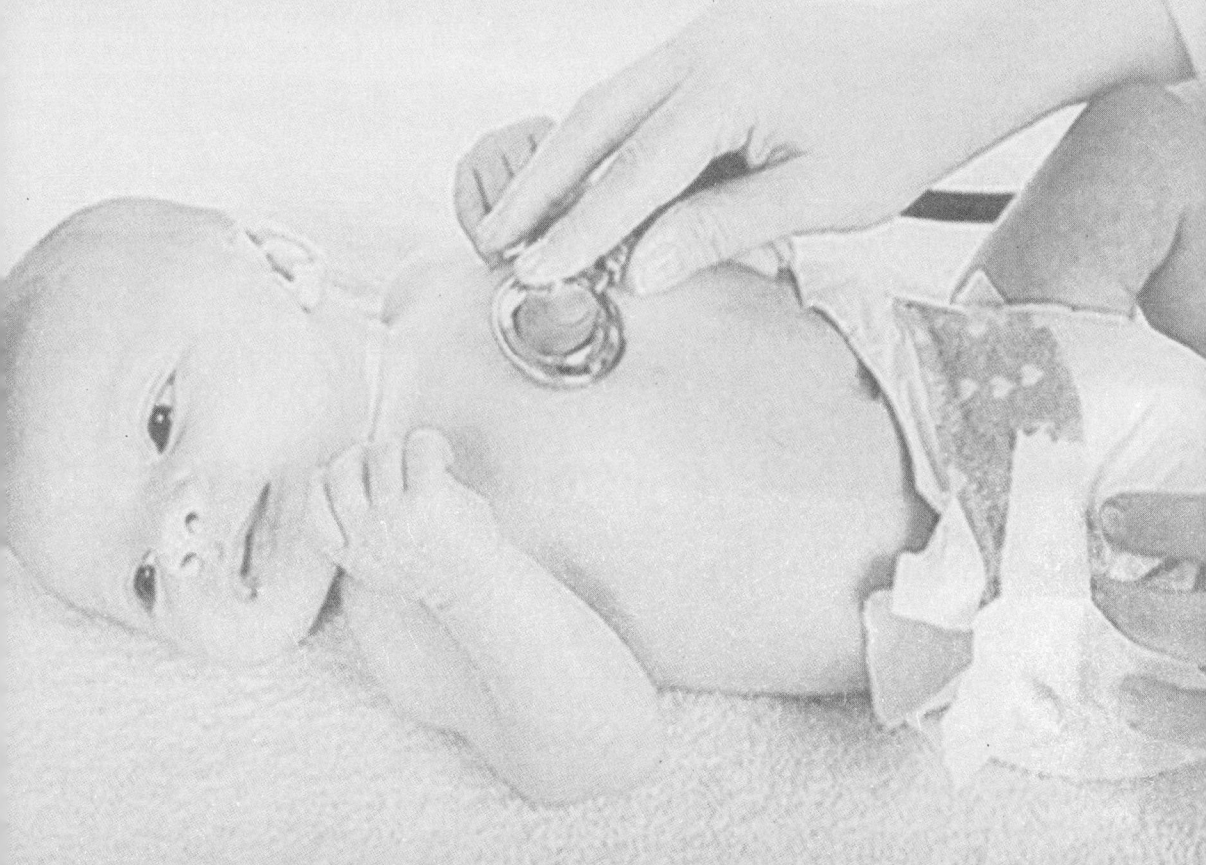

On the completion of this chapter, the pediatric nurse will be able to perform the following activity:
- Provide care to the baby through phototherapy

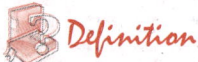 *Definition*

Phototherapy unit is a specially designed, electronically based instrument which has an effective light source for therapeutic purposes (Fig. 1).

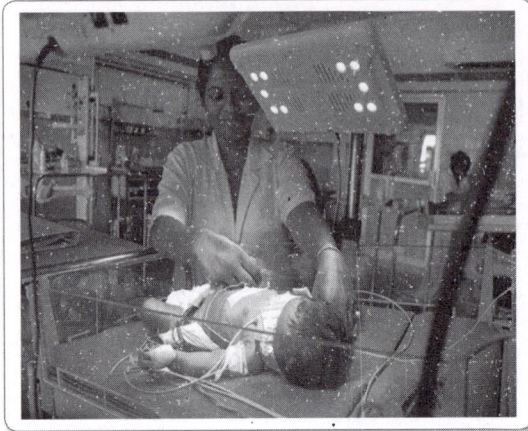

FIG. 1: Infant being given phototherapy

PURPOSE

This phototherapy unit is used to treat the neonatal jaundice by decreasing the serum bilirubin at normal range.

PARTS OF PHOTOTHERAPY UNIT

- Fluorescent lamp as a light source
- Side rails
- Platform to keep the baby
- Mattress (if single-layer phototherapy)
- Power cord for connecting with power supply
- On/off switch of light source
- Adjusting screw for light source.

TYPES

It is of two types—single-layer and double-layer phototherapy units.

ARTICLES NEEDED

- Cotton swab with sterile water or antiseptic solution to clean the phototherapy unit.
- Kidney tray or waste bin to discard the waste products.
- Eye shields/eye pads made up of cotton swab and gauze.
- Disposable napkin to cover the genitalia.
- Baby sheets.

CARE TO THE BABY

- Check the physician's orders and instructions.
- Wash your hands and clean the phototherapy unit with cotton swab properly.
- Check the phototherapy machine's working condition, e.g. bulbs, wires and electrical safety, power plug and power supply board. It should be free from sparking hazards. Advise the mother to feed the baby to prevent dehydration when exposed to phototherapy.
- Remove clothes of the baby and make the baby naked.
- Place the baby in the phototherapy unit.
- Apply the eye shield properly, which cover the both eyes.
- Cover the genitalia with napkin, which protects them from the lights.
- Side rails should be raised.
- Switch on the fluorescent lights and note the time.
- Continuously change the position, about every 2 hours, so that the lights reach all areas of the body.
- Record and report the observations.
- **Note:** Time of phototherapy care depends on the severity (level of bilirubin) of jaundice.
- Give the feeding at regular interval to maintain the fluid level.
- Change the napkin or diaper regularly.
- Do not give pressure over the eyes with eye shield.
- Continuously observe the skin for rashes, dryness etc.
- Do not apply oil to the skin of the baby because it can interfere with the effect of fluorescent lights.
- Observe side effects such as Bronze baby syndrome (greyish brown discolouration of skin and urine), skin rashes and loose green stool due to the increase in the bile flow.

MECHANISM OF ACTION

Fluorescent light of phototherapy unit breaks down the bilirubin. It acts by photo-oxidizing the tissue bilirubin and converts yellow lipid bilirubin into the colorless, nontoxic water-soluble bilirubin which can be easily excreted in the urine and bile.

13

Colostomy Care

- ➲ Introduction
- ➲ Purposes
- ➲ Indications
- ➲ Articles Needed
- ➲ Care and Procedure

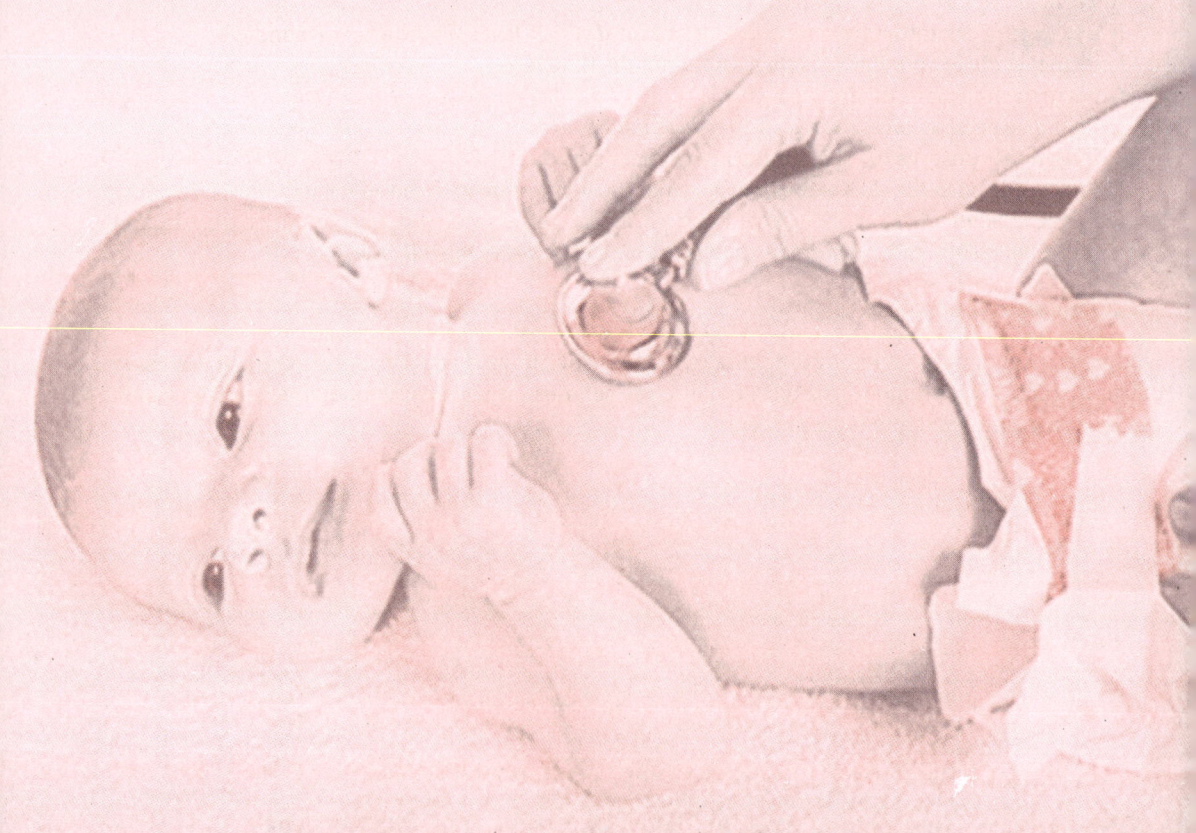

On the completion of this chapter, the pediatric nurse will be able to perform the following activities:
- Explain purposes of colostomy care
- Develop skills in care of the children with colostomy
- Inculcate these skills in their practical field.

INTRODUCTION

Colostomy care includes proper emptying of the colostomy bag and cleaning the colostomy site. Colostomy is a temporary or permanent opening of the colon on the anterior abdominal wall to permit the escape of faeces and flatus.

PURPOSES

- To prevent the excoriation of the skin around the stoma.
- To establish regularity of evacuation.
- To stop any leakage of feces.
- To teach the patient and parents/relatives regarding the care of the colostomy.

INDICATIONS

- It is used as a temporary measure to protect anastomosis.
- It is used for the newborn who have imperforate anus.
- It is used in cases of inflammatory/obstructive processes of the lower intestinal tract.

ARTICLES NEEDED

- Towel
- A pair of gloves
- Tissue paper
- Mackintosh with sheet
- Cotton swab and gauze pieces (Fig. 1)
- Soap and water
- Wash cloth
- Bed pan with the lid
- Disposable colostomy bag with clamp zinc oxide ointment.

CARE AND PROCEDURE

- Explain the procedure to the child and his or her parents.
- Keep all the equipment near the patient's side.
- Maintain a comfortable position, e.g. Fowler's, semi Fowler's position or sitting position in bathroom.
- Maintain privacy to the patient.
- Wash hands and wear the gloves.

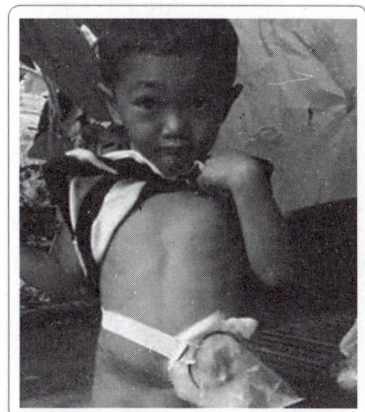

FIG. 1: Cover with gauze to prevent infection

- Empty the appliances and keep them in bedpan.
- Gradually remove the appliance, if the need arises. Use warm water to increase removal of appliance.
- Remove the excess stool with tissue paper from the stoma and keep stoma.
- Cover with gauze pad to prevent infection.
- Clean the peristomal skin with soap and water or any cleansing agent.
- If stoma is reddish pink in color, it indicates a normal condition.
- Now apply the zinc-oxide paste as skin barrier and keep it for 1–2 minutes to dry.
- Now apply the skin barrier and appliance together over the stoma.
- Remove the gauze pad covering the stoma.
- If required, instill deodorant in bag.
- Close the pouch if it is drainable with the clamp or clip.
- Discard the gloves and wastes and wash hands.
- Keep the stoma site dry to prevent infection.
- Recording and report the procedure.

14

Assisting in Exchange Transfusion

- ➲ Purposes
- ➲ Common Indications for Blood Transfusion
- ➲ Care and Procedure
- ➲ Complications of Blood Transfusion

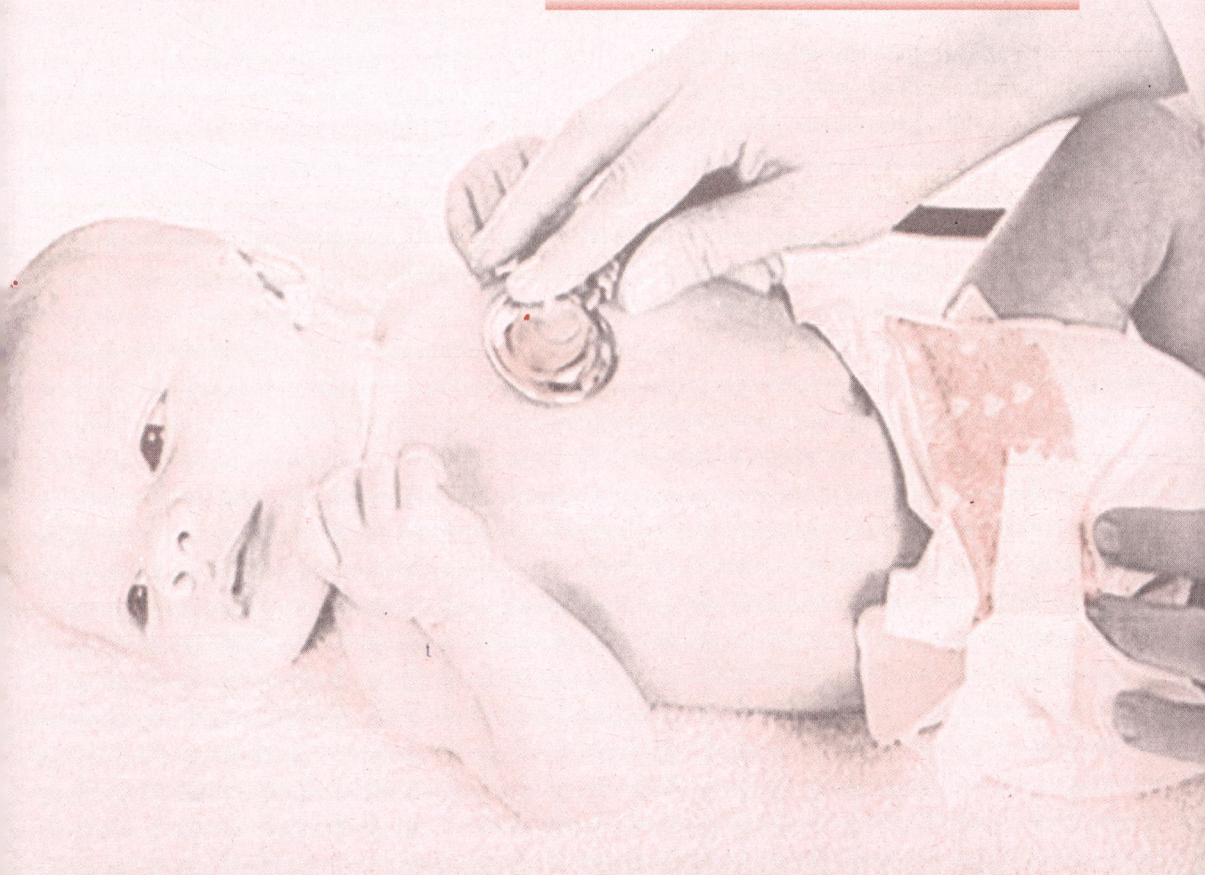

LEARNING OBJECTIVES

On the completion of this chapter, the pediatric nurse will be able to perform the following activities:
- Explain purposes and indication of blood transfusion
- Develop skills in assisting procedures
- Inculcate these skill in their practical field.

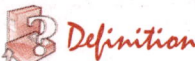 Definition

It is defined as assisting in exchange or replacement of blood in a newborn who is having Rh-positive blood from the Rh-negative mother and suffering from the hemolytic diseases.

PURPOSES

- To treat the anemia of children by replacing the Rh-positive red blood cells.
- To treat hyperbilirubinemia.
- To regulate blood volume.
- To remove the cells susceptible to hemolysis.

COMMON INDICATIONS FOR BLOOD TRANSFUSION

- When the cord blood hemoglobin level is less than 10 g/dL
- When cord blood bilirubin level is 5 mg/dL or more
- Increase in the reticulocytes
- When jaundice with serum bilirubin level is 20 mg/dL or more.

ARTICLES NEEDED

- Blood exchange transfusion kit containing: Bowel, kidney tray, suture scissors, toothed forceps, curved mosquito forceps, dressing forceps, surgical towel, syringes 10 and 20 cc, pads and bandages
- Dressing pack
- Sterile scalpel blade
- IV stand
- Injection: Heparin and normal saline
- Resuscitation equipment
- Oxygen source
- 3- or 4-way stopcock
- Umbilical vein catheter
- Gloves and masks
- Specimen containers
- Cord tie
- Scissors to cut the adhesive plaster
- Emergency drugs: Adrenalin, calcium gluconate, injection aminophylline
- Fresh blood for transfusion

CARE AND PROCEDURE

- Procedure should be properly explained to the parents and the caretaker.
- Take the informed written consent from the parent as per internationally accepted rights of children.
- The blood of donor should be cross-matched properly. Always use Rh-negative blood, and it is always preferable to use the same ABO group as the baby's.
- The blood should be fresh and not more than 5 days old.
- Maintain the nil per os (NPO) for about 4 hours before procedure.
- Immobilize the baby on cross splint.
- Clean umbilical stump by the dressing pack.
- The all apparatus should be primed with the saline and heparin injection in a bowl, to prevent stickiness.
- Now cut the umbilical cord less than 2.5 cm from the skin surface.
- Attach the ligature and insert the catheter into the vein.
- Fill the catheter with donor's blood before procedure to prevent from air embolism.
- Fix the catheter with an adhesive tape.
- Do the transfusion.
- Record the central venous pressure after the insertion of catheter.
- Check the vital signs and conditions of the baby.
- Test the blood samples after- and pre-procedure bloods to check the Hb level and bilirubin.
- Remove the catheter and give the cord tie at umbilicus, apply tincture benzoin at umbilicus and apply gauze and secure with adhesive tape.
- Keep the equipment properly after wash.
- Properly record and report.

Points to Remember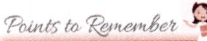

- Blood should be slowly warmed to the infant's body temperature.
- Fresh heparinized blood is used.
- About 20–30 mL of blood is withdrawn and about 10–20 mL blood is replaced each time.
- Place the baby in a radiant warmer after transfusion.
- Observe the umbilicus for finding the bleeding.

COMPLICATIONS OF BLOOD TRANSFUSION

- Umbilical vein perforation
- Cardiac arrest can occur
- Hypoglycemia and hypocalcemia
- Bacterial sepsis
- Metabolic acidosis
- Thrombocytopenia.

15

Respiratory Care

- ➲ Oxygen Therapy
- ➲ Tracheostomy Care
- ➲ Nebulization Therapy

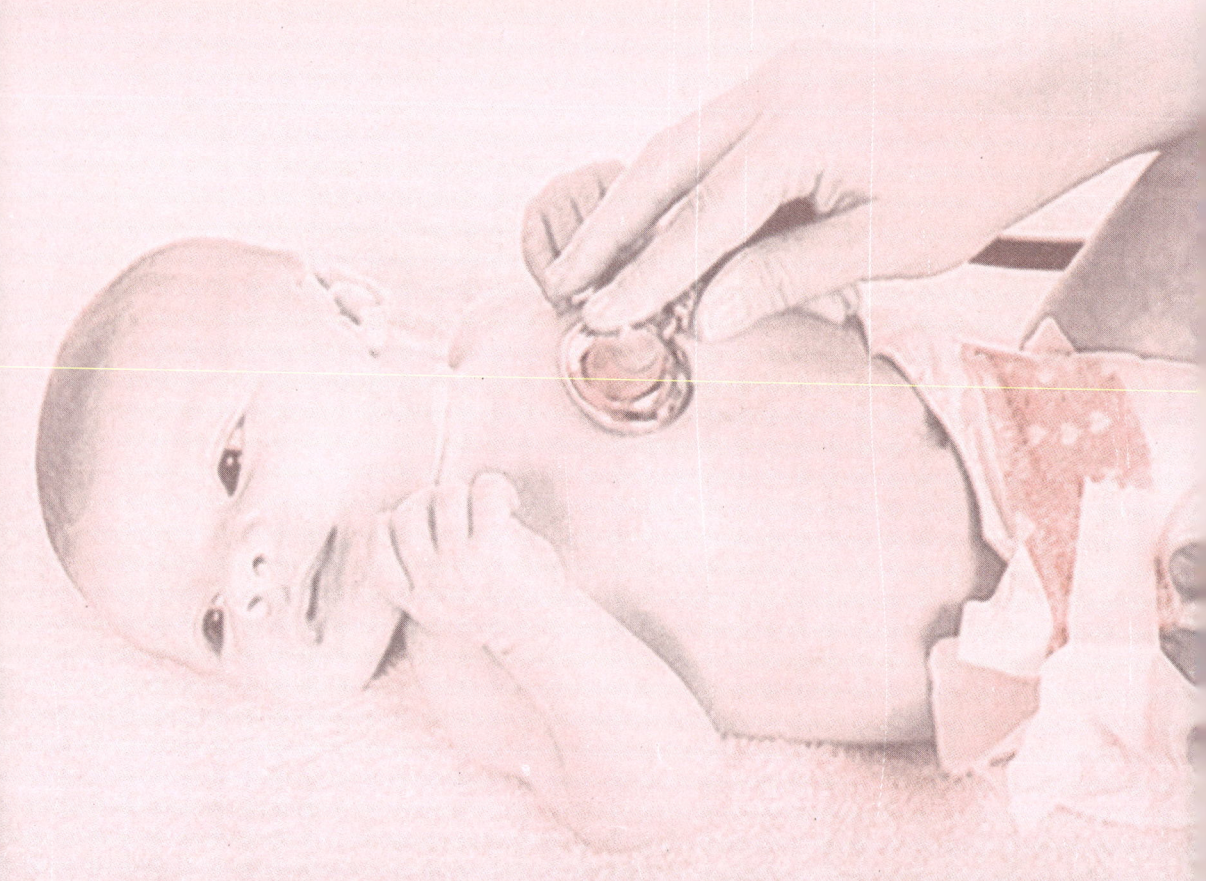

LEARNING OBJECTIVES

On the completion of this chapter, the pediatric nurse will be able to perform the following activities:
- Explain the methods and purposes of oxygen inhalation
- Develop skills in this procedure
- Inculcate these skills in their practical field
- Explain purposes and importance of nebulization
- Develop skills in this procedure
- Inculcate these skills in their practical field.

OXYGEN THERAPY

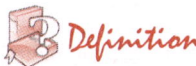
Definition

Administration of oxygen is a process of providing the O_2 supply to the child for the treatment of low concentration of O_2 in the blood. Children with respiratory dysfunctions are treated with oxygen inhalation to relieve anoxemia or hypoxemia (deficiency of oxygen in the blood). The normal amount of oxygen in the arterial blood should be in the range of 80–100 mm Hg. If it falls below 60 mm Hg, irreversible physiologic effects may occur. The oxygen administration treats the effects of oxygen deficiency but it does not correct the underlying causes.

Purposes

- To manage the condition of hypoxia.
- To maintain the oxygen tension in blood plasma.
- To increase the oxyhemoglobin in red blood cells.
- To maintain the ability of cells to carry out the normal metabolic function.
- To reduce the risk of complications.

Common Indications for Oxygen Administration

- **Cyanosis:** Bluish discoloration of skin, nail buds, mucus membranes, which result from a decreased amount of oxygen in the haemoglobin of the blood.
- **Breathlessness or labored breathing:** By some diseases such as emphysema, pulmonary embolism, coronary thrombosis etc.
- Anemia
- Diseases such as pulmonary edema, pneumonia, chest trauma, etc.
- Environment with low oxygen content, e.g. high attitudes.
- Poisoning with chemicals that alter the tissues, ability to utilize oxygen, e.g. cyanide poisoning.
- Hemorrhage
- Shock and circulatory failure.
- Children who are under anesthesia and critically ill.
- Asphyxia: Lack of oxygen by blocking the air passage such as drowning, foreign bodies, electrical shock, strangulations, etc.

Articles Needed

- Oxygen source: O_2 cylinder, central supply.
- Oxygen instrument according to methods such as oxygen mask, oxygen hood, nasal prongs, nasal catheter, oxygen tent or canopy.
- Humidifier
- Flow meter
- Gauze pieces
- Adhesive tape
- 'No smoking' signs
- Spinner to open the main valve of the oxygen cylinder
- Bowel with water to check the patency of the tube.

Methods of Oxygen Administration

Oxygen administration depends upon the condition of the child, age, desired concentration facilities available and the preference of the doctor. Oxygen administration can be given continuously or intermittently. It depends on the requirement of the child. It is given in 40–60% concentration. Following are the methods of oxygen administration:

- **Administration of O_2 by nasal catheter:** This is a very common method of O_2 administration in hospital settings. A catheter is inserted into the nostril reaching up to the uvula and is held in place by adhesive tapes. This catheter does not interfere with the child's freedom to eat, to talk and to move on the bed. Catheter nos. 4–6 are used and it should be 7.5–10 cm inserted in the nasopharynx. The catheter should be removed every 8 hours, and a new catheter should be inserted by using other nostril alternatively. The catheter method is used for the older children. The amount of oxygen should be 4 liter per minute.

- **Administration of oxygen by the mask:** Today, there are various face masks available that cover the child's mouth and nose for O_2 administration. The mask size should match child's size. It should be properly fitted, and if it does not fit properly, O_2 will be lost from the mask. It should be removed after every 4 hours and the face should be wiped. The masks are advantageous patients who are unable to breathe through the nose. The flow of oxygen should be about 2–3 liter for young children and 1–2 liter/minute for the infants.

- **Administration of oxygen by the tent method:** This method consists of a canopy over the patient's bed, that covers the patient fully or partially. The oxygen tent is made up of plastic material, transparent to prevent absorption of oxygen. The lower part of the canopy is tucked under the bed to prevent the escape of oxygen. There are certain advantages and disadvantages for using a oxygen tent method.

Advantages

- Oxygen tent provides the environment for the patient with controlled oxygen concentration, temperature regulation and humidity control.
- It allows freedom for free movement in bed.

Disadvantages

- It creates a feeling of isolation.

- It requires high volume of oxygen, which is not easily available.
- When the tent is opened, there is loss of O_2 concentration.
- It has more chances of fire.
- It requires more time and cleanliness to maintain a tent.

Complications of O_2 Administration

- **Infection:** By using the contaminated equipment, the causative organisms can be present in such places as tracheostomy or endotracheal tubes, catheters, humidifying water and masks etc.
- **Drying of mucus membrane of the respiratory tract:** It can occur when oxygen is administered without sufficient humidity. It can cause irritation and drying of the mucous membrane.
- **Combustion (fire):** O_2 itself does not burn, but it supports combustion.
- **Oxygen toxicity:** Symptoms of toxicity includes tracheal irritation and cough.
- **Atelectasis:** Collapse of alveoli develops as a result of increased oxygen concentration in the inspired air. This is due to elimination of nitrogen.
- **Oxygen-induced apnea:** The carbon dioxide is washed off completely from the blood by a high concentration of oxygen. The respiratory centre is not stimulated sufficiently.
- **Asphyxia :** Patients who receive O_2 by masks and close tents must be protected from asphyxia.
- **Retrolental fibroplasias:** The hazards of oxygen may affect the eyes. It is noted in premature infants who have a high concentration of oxygen inhalation.
- Some other complications are bronchopulmonary, dysplasia, respiratory depression, seizure disorders and epilepsy.

Important Instruction for Oxygen Inhalation

- Oxygen should be prescribed in specific dose. It acts as a drug and causes oxygen toxicity.
- Always use humidifier and regulator.
- All the articles should be cleaned and a disposable nasal catheter should be used and the nasal catheter should be changed every 8 hours.
- Lubricate the nasal catheter before inserting.
- Control valve of cylinder should be adjusted only when catheter is out of nose, or during oxygenation, do not alter the valve.
- Discontinue the oxygen gradually.
- Leave a calling signal or bell near the patient while going away from the patient.
- Keep in close observation conditions, which can interfere with the flow of oxygen from the source to the patient.
- Keep ready one cylinder to prevent the deprivation of oxygen.
- Give oxygen in low concentration to the premature babies to prevent the retrolental fibroplasia.
- Continuously monitor the patient to find out the oxygen toxicity symptoms.
- Empty cylinder should marked "empty" and kept separately from full cylinders.
- While oxygen administration, paste the "No Smoking" signs near the patient's bed or on the door.
- Record and report the observations property.

Procedure

- Ensure all the parts are available

- Ensure oxygen cylinder is secured on flat surface in a trolley. There is no naked flame nearby and do not use oil/greese to lubricate the joints
- Attach the regulator
- Attach flow meter to the regulator to set the flow rate. Ensure the flow meter is vertical
- Attach humidification bottle to the flow meter. Fill clean water up to the mark level on the bottle. Ensure the humidifier bottle is washed daily with soap and water and water is changed daily.
- Attach an oxygen tube to the humidifier
- Using a spanner/key, turn on oxygen from the cylinder and set the desired flow rate from the flow meter. Ensure there are no leaks
- Connect oxygen tube to the nasal prongs/catheter/face mask/oxygen hood to deliver oxygen to the patient
- Ensure the nose is clear. Place the nasal prongs just inside the nostril. Run the tubing under the nostril alongside the child's head and tape's it, adjust the oxygen flow rate at 0.5–1 litre per minute for children less than 2 months and 1–2 litre per minute for children 2 months up to 5 years

TRACHEOSTOMY CARE

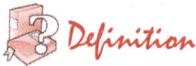 Definition

It is a surgical procedure in which an opening is made in the trachea to enable the patient to breathe.

Indications

- Laryngotracheobronchitis
- Epiglotitis with edema or laryngeal spasm
- Foreign bodies that cannot be removed via larynx
- Congenital anomalies
- Central nervous system disorders
- Subglottic stenosis
- Tracheomalacia
- Vocal cord paralysis

Articles Needed

A sterile tray containing
- Tracheostomy tube
- Obturator and extra inner cannula
- Tracheostomy ties
- Small curved scissors
- Blunt hemostat
- Cotton tipped applicators
- Water
- 3% hydrogen peroxide
- Betadine swab

- Dressing pads
- Oxygen
- Self inflating resuscitation bag
- Lubricating jelly
- Call bell within the child's reach
- Suction equipment
  - A pair of sterile gloves
  - Suction apparatus with good negative pressure
  - Sterile suction catheters
- No 6 Fr. catheters for infants and young children and No 8–10 for old children
  - Sterile saline

Preparation of Child and Family

- Explain the procedure and its indications
- Tracheostomy care procedure
  - Position the child supine with a blanket or towel roll to extend the neck
  - Open all packaging and cut tracheostomy ties to appropriate length if necessary
  - Clean around the tracheostomy site with antiseptic solution
  - Rinse with sterile water and cotton tipped applicator in similar fashion
  - Place the pre-cut sterile gauze under the tracheostomy tube
  - With the assistant holding the tube in place, cut the ties and remove the tube
  - Attach the clean ties to the tube and secure in a safe place.

Points to Remember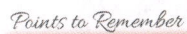

Nurse's Responsibility in Care of Tracheostomy
- The child with tracheostomy is placed in an area of high visibility
- Children normally communicate their needs by crying but the tracheostomy prohibits vocalization
- Maintain patency of the tube

Suction Depths

- Shallow suctioning
- Premeasured suctioning
- Deep suctioning

Care Techniques

- Sterile technique
- Modified sterile suctioning technique
- Clean technique

Procedure

- Explain the procedure
- Wash hands
- Set up equipment and connect suction catheter to machine tubing

- Pour normal saline into cup
- Put on gloves
- Turn on suction machine
- Place tip of the catheter into a saline cup to moisten and to see that suction is working
- Use saline only if the mucus is very thick, hard to cough up or difficult to suction.
- Gently insert the catheter into the trach tube without applying suction.
- Put thumb over opening in catheter to create suction and use a circular motion while withdrawing the catheter so that the mucus is removed well from all areas. Avoid suctioning longer than 10 seconds because of oxygen loss.

Nurse's Responsibility in Suctioning

- When suctioning, do not apply suction as the catheter is introduced.
- Withdraw the catheter while rotating and applying suction by covering the part on the catheter with the thumb.
- Hold the suction for no more than 5 seconds.
- The child should be allowed to rest for about a minute and take two or three breaths between suctioning.
- Hyperventilate the child with 100% oxygen.
- Change the position frequently.
- Careful bathing to prevent water entering the tube.
- Fowler's position is preferred during feeding.
- Trachties: Antibiotic apply on skin breakdown under the trachties
- Suction pressure
  - Infant 60: 100 mm Hg
  - Children: 100–110 mm Hg
  - Adult: 110–150 mm Hg
- Chest physiotherapy can be given to remove the secretions.

Complications

- Haemorrhage
- Wound infection
- Atelectasis
- Death

NEBULIZATION THERAPY

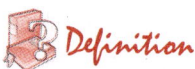 Definition

It is a therapy which is used to treat the respiratory problem or a method of treatment for patient with respiratory infection by an electronic device known as nebulizer which is used for spraying the medications into the deeper part of respiratory tract in the form of cloud-like fine particles or fine mist (vapour).

Nebulizer and its Parts

It is an electronic device or a machine that sprays medicine into the respiratory tract in the form of fine mist. It is also known as 'breathing machine.' A nebulizer has the following parts:

- Compressor
- Lid
- Air outlet connector
- Power switch (on–off)
- Carrying handle
- Filter for air
- Power cord
- Power cord storage recess
- Nebulizer air inlet connector
- Medication cup/nebulizer cup
- Cap or dome
- Baffle
- Mouth piece adult/child
- Face mask adult/child
- Tubing
- Accessories storage recess

Purpose

- To treat the condition of respiratory tract by adding airborne water particles
- To thin the secretion
- Induce a productive cough
- In conditions of pneumonia, asthma, cough, bronchiectasis etc.
- To deposit pharmacologic agent in upper and lower airways
- Sputum induction
- It is also given immediately before bronchial drainage to increase the effectiveness of the procedure
- To decrease bronchial oedema

Why do we Need the Nebulizer?

It sends the medicine directly into the deeper part of the lungs and the effect is more and the patient can get better faster (Fig. 1).

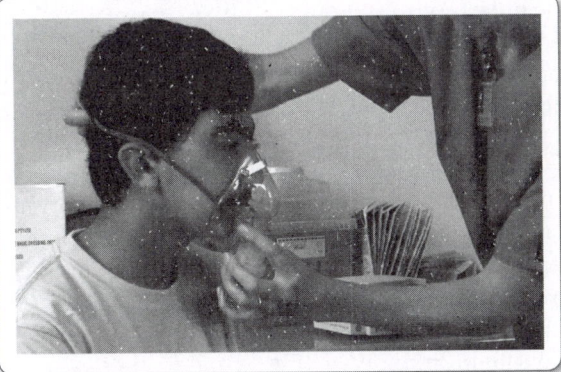

FIG. 1: Nebulization given to a patient

Indications

- Children with acute respiratory tract infections
- Children with asthma, pneumonia, cough, bronchiectasis etc.

Contraindication

Child with history of hypersensitivity

Complications

- Can irritate the mucosa and can cause bronchospasm and dyspnoea
- Infection from the contaminated equipment
- Over hydration
- Over mobilisation of secretions
- Blockage of gas flow to the patient by fluid accumulation in tubing
- Adverse reaction from medication

Prevention of Complications

- By proper cleaning of the instruments and articles
- By administration of proper drug therapy
- Follow-up care as ordered by the paediatrician.

Drugs Used for Nebulization Therapy

- Mucolytic drugs
- Decongestant drugs
- Bronchodilators

Antimicrobial Agents

The following drugs are available as inhalation for nebulization:
- Salbutamol (Asthalin respirator solution)
- Terbutaline (Bricanyl nebulization solution)
- Salmeterol (Solvent solution)
- Beclomethasone (Beclate)
- Budesonide (Budecort, pulmicort respules)
- Ipratropium (Ipravent solution)

Asthalin Respirator Solution

This is the commonly used medicine or drug to treat the respiratory disorders which contains salbutamol (bronchodilator). The dilution of medicine drugs and therapy depends on the doctor's order. The explaining preparation of medicine should be in the following ratio:

Adult: 0.5 to 1 mL (2.5 to 5 mg) +2 to 4 mL normal saline or distilled water. **Child:** Up to 3 years: 0.1 mL (Asthalin solution) + 2 mL normal saline 3 to 12 years 0.5 mL (Asthalin solution) +2 mL normal saline.

Frequency: 6 hourly or 8 hourly

Duration: 10–15 minutes, average 10 minutes.

How Does the Aerosol Mist Enter into the Lungs?

As the patient inhales, the fine mist passes from the mouth, nose through the wind pipe (trachea) into a system of airway (bronchus) that divides into smaller (lobar bronchus) units and then segmental bronchus divides into bronchioles, bronchioles divides into the respiratory bronchioles. The respiratory bronchioles carries aerosol (fine mist) into the tiny air sacs, alveoli through the alveolar duct, where gas exchange takes place and fine mist produces its effect.

Articles Needed

A tray containing the following articles:
- Nebulizer machine/compressor with all accessories
- Sputum cup: For taking the cough while child feels coughing
- Kidney tray: For discarding the dirty swabs
- A bowl with spirit-soaked cotton swabs
- A bowl with dry sterile cotton swabs
- Surgical spirit for disinfection
- Stethoscope: To auscultate the breath sound
- Face towel: For wiping the face if perspiration is present.
- Hand towel: For wiping the hands
- Medicine: Respiratory solution (prescribed by the paediatrician)
- Dropper or disposal syringe: To pour the medicine in the medicine cup
- Additional set of face mask, tube and medication chamber
- A ball pen: To enter the procedure in the nurse's record
- Watch: To note the time duration for nebulization therapy.

Procedure

Pre-Procedure

- Wash the hands before doing the procedure and explain the procedure to the parents
- Select a suitable place to administer nebulization therapy.
- Clean and wipe the nebulizer and its accessories and check whether the nebulizer is in working condition.
- Check and assemble all the articles at the bedside of the child.
- Pour prescribed medicine in correct dilution in the nebulizer cup and tightly cover it with a dome.
- Provide Fowler's position to the child and auscultate the child for breath sound (pit observation).
- Place the face mask, which cover the nose and mouth, and instruct the child to take deep breath.

During the Procedure

- Switch on the nebulizer and observe the patency of the tube which is connected to the nebulizer.
- Administer nebulization therapy for 10–15 minutes and observe the child for any side effects and note the time of starting the therapy.
- Turn off the nebulizer when the patient's treatment is over or while the child feels coughing.

After the Procedure

- Provide the child a comfortable position and encourage to cough out.
- Check the breath sound of the child by auscultation (postobservation)

- If perspiration is present, wipe the child's face with clean soft face towel.
- Wash and replace all the articles and keep them ready for the next use.
- Record the procedure and vital signs in nurse's notes and report to the staff nurse in charge.

Cleaning the Nebulizer and its Accessories

If the nebulizer is not cleaned it might pick up germs and cause the cross-infection to another child.

How to Clean?

- After each use, the device must be cleaned.
- Disassemble the mouth piece, nose piece or face mask from cap, open nebulizer cup and remove baffle.
- Wash all the items, except tubing in a hot water/detergent solution, rinse under the hot tap water remove detergent residue. Allow to air dry on clean paper.
- Keep the outer surface of the tubing dust free by wiping regularly with the clean dry cotton swab once in a day. Nebulizer tubing does not have to be washed because only filtered air passes through it.
- Use a dry clean cloth to clean the outer part of the nebulizer.

Compressor Cleaning

- With power switch in the 'off' position, unplug the power cord from wall outlet.
- Wipe outside of the compressor cabinet with a clean damp cloth or dry cotton to keep dust free.

Points to Remember

Important Safeguards
- The nebulizer must not be touched with wet or soaked hands.
- No smoking or no sparks around the electrical equipment.
- Do not submerge the nebulizer in water; doing so will result in damage to the compressor.
- Do not pour medication solution more than 10 mL into the jet nebulizer/medication cup.
- Filter should be changed every month or sooner if it turns completely grey. Do not wash or clean the filter.
- Do not dry the nebulizer parts with a towel; this could contaminate them.
- Completely dry the nebulizer after use and store all its accessories in a clean, dry and safe area.

16

Care of Child on Ventilator

- ⊃ Indications for Mechanical Ventilation
- ⊃ Modes of Mechanical Ventilation
- ⊃ Types of Ventilators
- ⊃ Ways of Delivery of Gas through Mechanical Ventilation
- ⊃ Care and Monitoring of the Ventilated Child

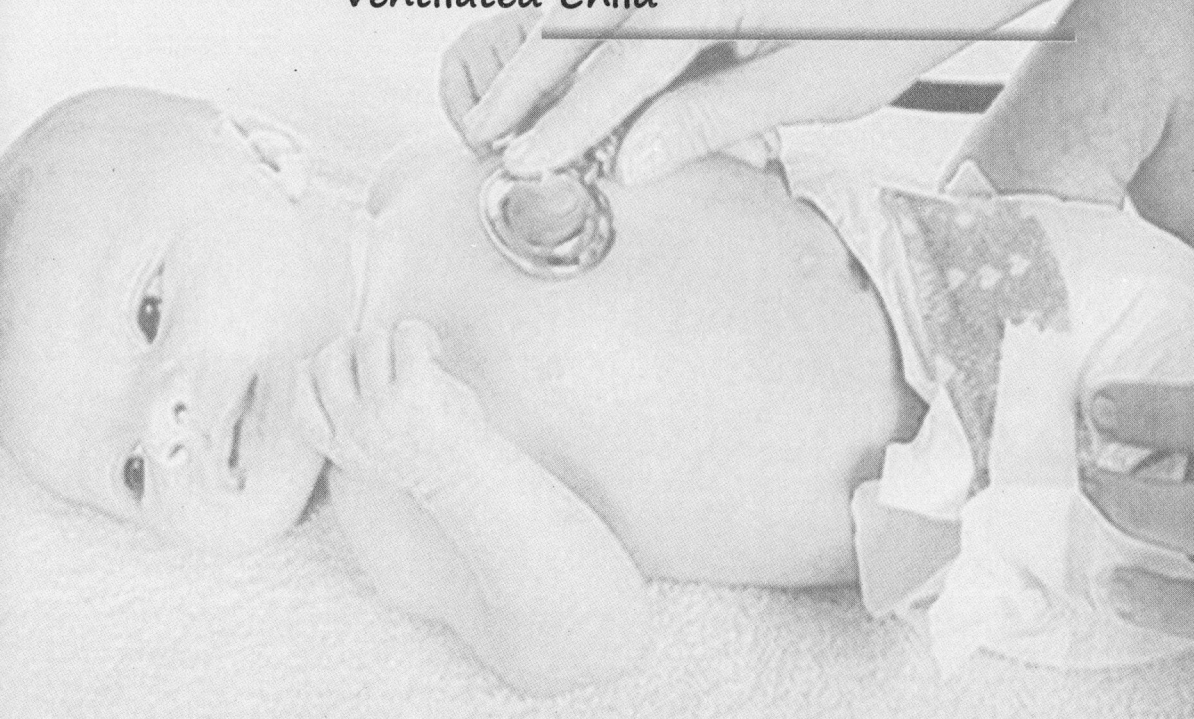

LEARNING OBJECTIVES

On completion of this chapter, the pediatric nurse will be able to perform the following activities:
- Explain the purpose of ventilator
- Identify the indications
- List the different modes of ventilation
- Develop the skill in care of child on ventilation
- Inculcate the skills in their practical field

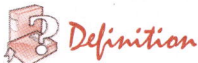 *Definition*

Ventilation may be defined as the movement of air in and out of the lungs. Respiration is defined as the process of gas exchange within the lungs (external) or at the tissue level (internal). It may be spontaneous or assisted.

Assisted ventilation involves an external device connected directly to the patient which provides the movements of air in and out of the lungs. This device may be a resuscitative bag or a mechanical ventilator.

Ventilator is an electronically based device which is used to assist or replace the work of the respiratory muscles and the thorax to maintain the gas exchange function of the lungs. These are also known as mechanical ventilators.

INDICATIONS FOR MECHANICAL VENTILATION

- Respiratory failure resulting due to pulmonary disease, apnea caused by the central nervous system pathology or injury, infections
- Respiratory muscle weakness
- Neuromuscular disease or chest wall trauma
- Foreign body obstruction
- Medication toxicity
- Inadequate respiration effort
- Excessive work of breathing, manifested by retractions, tachypnea and decreasing O_2 saturation.

MODES OF MECHANICAL VENTILATION

There are following modes of ventilation:
- **Controlled ventilation:** In controlled ventilation, all the breaths are triggered, limited and cycled by the ventilator. This mode is used when the patient's ventilator drive is limited or absent or has been suppressed using drugs or when the patient has been paralyzed.
- **Assisted ventilation:** Assisted ventilation reduces the patient's effort and optimizes comfort. This ventilation is identical to the controlled mode except that the patient's inspiratory effort triggers the ventilator to deliver the breath using preselected limit and cycle variables, and the ventilator completes the rest.
- **Supported ventilation:** It is defined as the breaths that are triggered by the patient, limited by the ventilator and cycled by the patient.

TYPES OF VENTILATORS

There are three major types:

- **Pressure-cycled ventilator:** This type of ventilator terminates the respiratory cycle when a preset inspiratory pressure is reached. Volume will differ greatly, depending on the flow rate of the delivery of the gas. The compliance of the lung will affect the tidal volume even though the pressure will remain constant.
- **Volume-cycled ventilator:** This type of ventilator terminates respiration when a present volume (tidal volume) is delivered. The compliance and resistance of the lung will change the pressure needed to deliver the preset volume.
- **Time-cycled ventilator:** This type of ventilator terminates inspiration when a preset time is reached. Tidal volume is greatly affected by the compliance of the ventilator tubing, compliance and resistance of the lung and flow rate of the delivered gas. The duration of the inspiratory pressure will be affected by the preset inspiratory time and flow rate of the delivered gas.

WAYS OF DELIVERY OF GAS THROUGH MECHANICAL VENTILATION

Mechanical ventilation may deliver a volume of gas to the patient's lungs in one of these following two ways:

- **Positive pressure ventilation (PPV):** Positive pressure is applied directly to the airway, which forces air down the airways and into the lungs.
- **Negative pressure ventilation (NPV):** Negative pressure is applied externally to the chest cage, which will change the pressure dynamics so that the gas flows from the relatively positive atmosphere to the relatively negative air spaces. Both the techniques may be used in the pediatric ventilation although PPV is more common today.

CARE AND MONITORING OF THE VENTILATED CHILD

- During mechanical ventilation, the caregiver or nurse has to take a huge responsibility.
- Close monitoring of all the vitals of the patient should be done.
- The nutrition should meet the total nutrition requirements; for example, calorie and protein requirements must be completed.
- Excessive carbohydrate should be avoided as it may result in increased CO_2 production.
- Before use of medications to sedate the child, it should be ensured that the ET tube is patent, in good position and well secured.
- Check that ventilator setting should be appropriate and no complications should occur.
- Assess frequency and strength of spontaneous breathing.
- Observe the chest wall inflation and frequency of air entry/exit.
- Monitoring of circulation—pulse and blood pressure should be done.
- Abdominal distension should be done.
- Assess neurobehavioral activity.
- Radiological assessment should be performed.
- Monitor position of ET tube, and nasogastric tube.
- Overall lung volume should be assessed.
- Monitor any air leak syndrome—emphysema, pneumothorax, etc.
- Presence of atelectasis, pneumonia, pulmonary edema, etc should be checked.
- Check heart size or any complications.

17

Assess the Child with Special Diagnostic Approach

- ➲ MRI
- ➲ Lumbar Puncture
- ➲ Liver Biopsy
- ➲ Renal Biopsy
- ➲ Bone Marrow Aspiration
- ➲ Needle Biopsy

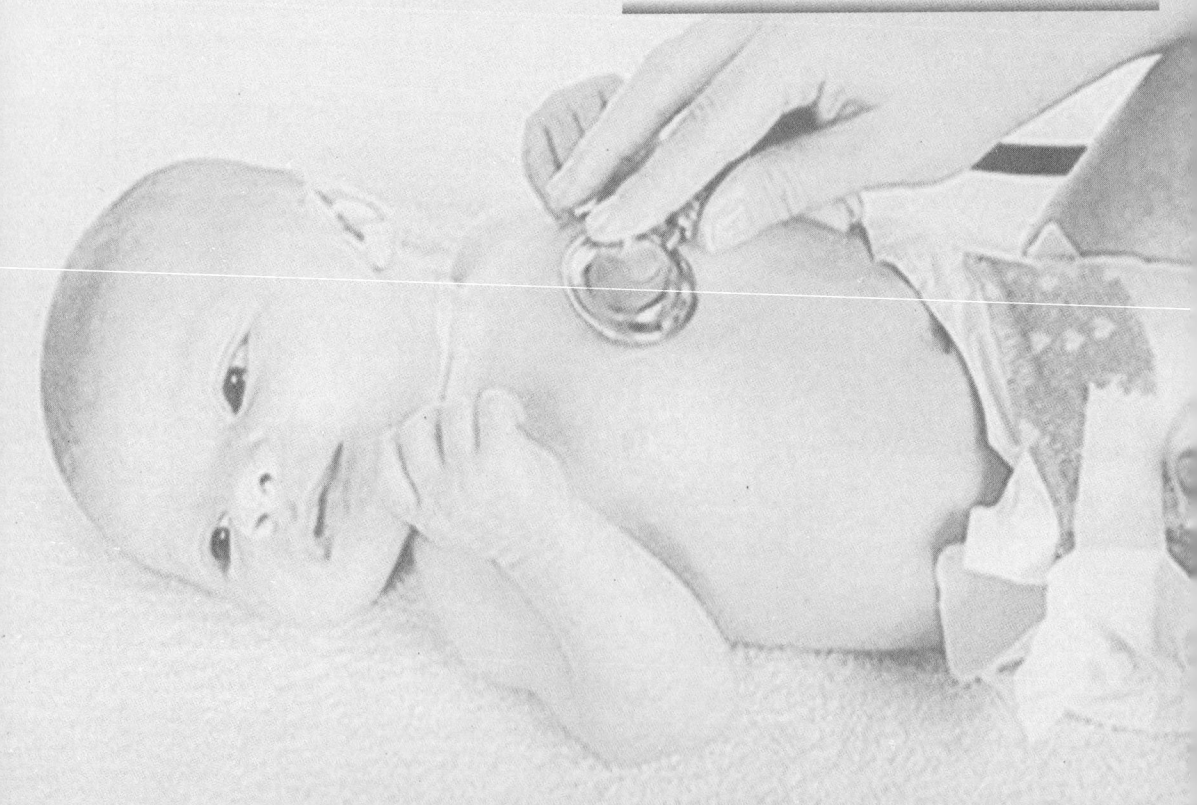

LEARNING OBJECTIVES

On the completion of this chapter, the pediatric nurse will be able to perform the following activities:
- Explain purposes of MRI
- Identify indications
- Manage the pre-and postpreparation of child for MRI
- Develop skill on this procedure
- Inculcate the skill in their practical field
- Perform lumbar puncture
- Perform renal biopsy and liver biopsy
- Perform bone marrow aspiration
- Explain the preparation of child for needle biopsy
- Develop the skill in care of child for needle biopsy
- Inculcate the skill in their practical field.

MRI

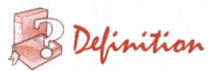 *Definition*

It is a medical technique used in radiology to investigate the anatomy and physiology of the body in both health and disease. MRI scanners use strong magnetic fields and radio waves to form images of the body.

PURPOSES

- To diagnose diseases of the central nervous system including the brain and the spine.
- To detect musculoskeletal disorders and injuries.
- To identify complications of infectious diseases such as AIDS.
- To determine medical diagnosis, staging of cancer and follow-up without exposure to ionizing radiation.
- To image the cardiovascular system.
- To detect congenital heart defect in neonates.
- To evaluate bone marrow disease.
- To assist in the planning of surgery and cancer treatment.
- To evaluate the traumatic injury, speech delay, creatine deficiency syndrome, mood disorder in young children.

PRECAUTIONS

- Prior to the procedure, patients are required to remove all the metal objects and remove any clothing with metal on them.
- In most cases, parents need to complete a survey regarding their child's past surgical and medical history to indicate whether the child has any metallic implants.
- Avoid MRI with metallic implants that include artificial joints, pacemakers, aneurysm, pins or screws and staples.

- During the examination, the child must lie still. The MRI scanner does make loud noises throughout the examination, which can be frightening for some children.
- Before the examination, the procedure should be explained to the child and it should be emphasised that the examination is painless.

PROCEDURE

- Children undergoing an MRI scan are appropriately positioned on the patient table by the technologist.
- For some scans, an injectable contrast media may be used and is administered using an intravenous catheter.
- Once the patient is positioned, the technologist goes to an adjacent control room to operate the scanner.
- The technologist uses an intercom system to instruct the child to hold their breath or remain still at certain times during the scan.
- Scan ranges from 30 to 90 minutes depending on the type of scan.
- When the MRI machine scans, the child hears loud, clanging and whirring noises.
- To alleviate the fear or stress related to hearing this noise and being inside the small scanning tools, the child may be offered earplugs or specially designed headphones for listening to music.

AFTERCARE

- No special aftercare is required following MRI scans unless sedation or general anesthesia was used during the scan.
- The children are required to remain in a supervised recovery area for an hour or more following to monitor for reaction to anaesthesia.

RISKS

- Some children and adolescents may feel claustrophobic.
- Younger infants and children have headache and vomiting.

PARENTAL CONCERN

- Younger children may be frightened of the MRI scanner and might require the presence of a parent or other family members in the scanning room.
- To help alleviate fear, taking the child into the MRI room to see the equipment prior to the procedure may be helpful.

LUMBAR PUNCTURE (FIG. 1)

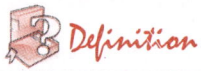 Definition

A lumbar puncture (LP), often called a spinal tap, is a common medical test that involves taking a small sample of cerebrospinal fluid (CSF) for examination. CSF is a clear, colorless liquid that delivers nutrients and "cushions" the brain and spinal cord, or central nervous system.

STEPS OF PROCEDURE

- Obtain an informed consent.
- Gather materials.
- Position the patient.
- Administer local anaesthetic.
- Insert the needle with sterile technique.
- Measure the opening pressure.
- Collect cerebrospinal fluid (CSF).
- Send to lab.
- Care of articles and child.
- Documentation.

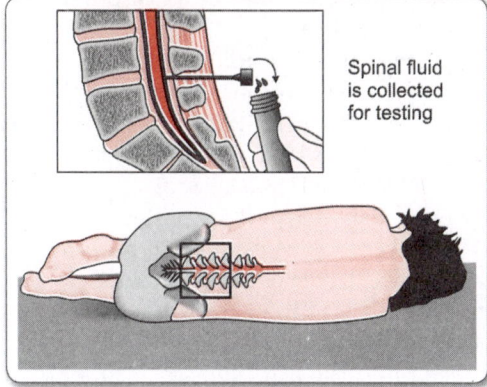

Spinal fluid is collected for testing

FIG. 1: Lumbar puncture

Informing the Patient

- **Reason for the lumbar puncture:**
  Collection and testing of spinal fluid are standard management for encephalitis patients to direct treatment (e.g., if CSF profile suggests bacterial infection).

Potential Complications

- The most common side effect is a headache which occurs in 10–30% of adult patients. It is managed with bed rest and analgesics and usually disappears in a few days.
- Soreness of the lower back may also occur.
- Other risks, including infection, bleeding, leakage of spinal fluid or damage to the spinal cord are extremely rare.
- Children tolerate lumbar punctures really well.

Articles Needed

- Clean trolley
- Masks—for person performing procedure and assistant
- Sterile gown pack
- Sterile gloves
- Sterile plastic drape
- Sterile scissors
- Basic dressing pack
- Antiseptic solution as per unit protocol
- Ampoule of sterile water
- Lumbar puncture needle—short bevel, 22 or 25 gauge.
- 23 or 25 g needles are occasionally used by experienced practitioners when a lumbar puncture cannot be satisfactorily achieved with a standard LP needle.
- Sterile pack of 3 CSF collection tubes (Fig. 2)

Position for Lumbar Puncture (Fig. 3)

- Place the Patient in the Left Lateral Position

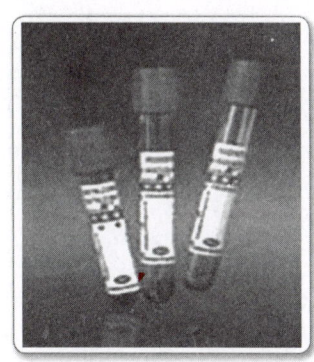

FIG. 2: Park of 3 CSF collection tubes

- The lower back should be as close to the edge of the bed as possible.
- Ask the patient to curl up and hug his knees as close to the chest as possible ("fetal position").
- The neck should be flexed forward.
- If physician is left-handed, the right lateral position should be used.
- The patient may also be positioned sitting upright. However, the lateral position is preferred for accurate measurement of opening pressure.

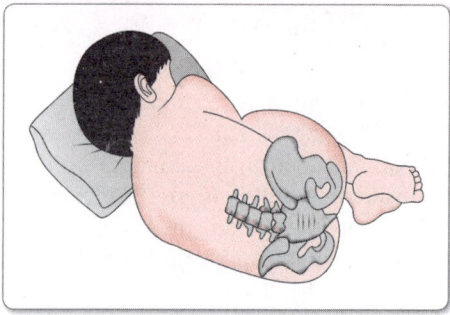

FIG. 3: Lumbar puncture position

Locate the Site

- Find and palpate the posterior iliac crest.
- Move your finger down and palpate the L4 spinous process.
- Mark the puncture site at L4-5 or L3-4 [e.g. put a slight indent in the skin with your fingernail (Figs 4 and 5)].

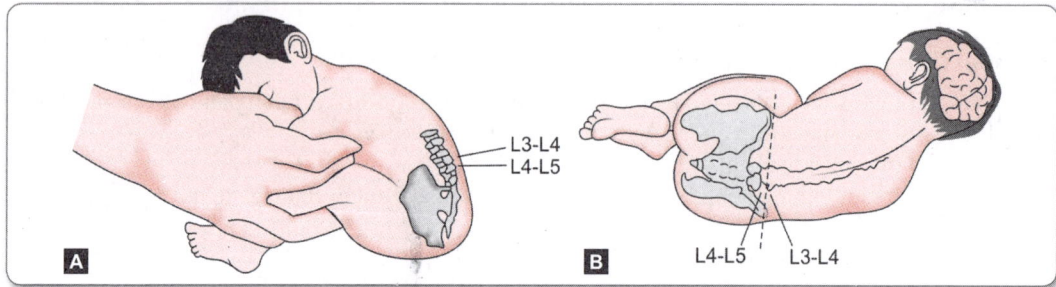

FIGS 4A AND B: **A.** Site for lumbar puncture in a child; **B.** Having the patient curl around a pillow can help ensure proper position

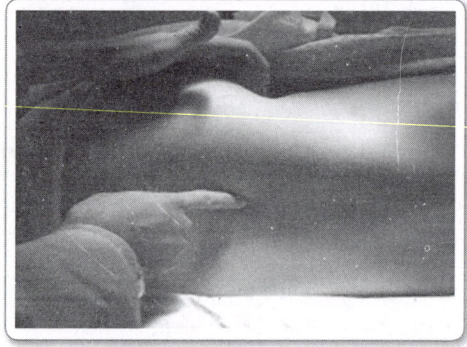

FIG. 5: Indicating site of posterior iliac crest and puncture site

Prepare Sterile Area

- Use iodine to swab in a circle from the L4-5 area outwards.
- Cover an area of 20 cm diameter (Fig. 6).

- Once dried, remove the iodine with alcohol (to avoid introduction of iodine into the subarachnoid space).

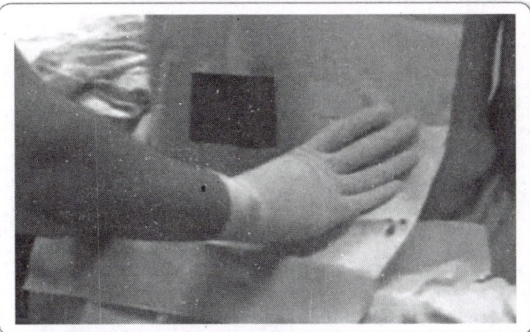

FIG. 6: Cover the area

Anaesthetize the Area

- Anaesthetize the skin.
- Anaesthetize between the spinous processes.
  - Insert the needle.
  - Draw back to ensure it has not reached the subarachnoid space.
  - Gradually withdraw the syringe while slowly injecting anaesthetic into the interspace.

Insert the Lumbar Puncture Needle

- Insert the LP needle with the stylet in the midline.
- Direct the point of the needle to the umbilicus.
- Keep the needle parallel to the ground.
- Continue to insert until a slight pop is felt.
- Withdraw the stylet slightly to ensure that the needle is in the subarachnoid space.
- If there is no CSF return, advance the needle about 2–3 mm, and withdraw the stylet again.
- When CSF begins to flow, attach a three-way stop–cock.

Notes on LP Needle Insertion
- If the needle strikes bone, withdraw it to just below the skin, then reinsert.
- If blood slowly drips from the needle when the stylet is removed, discard the needle and start again.
- Never aspirate CSF with a syringe, as a nerve root may be trapped against the needle and injured.
- If you are unsuccessful in reaching subarachnoid space, check:
  - Is the needle aimed towards the umbilicus?
  - Is the needle in the midline?
  - Is the needle parallel to the ground?

Measure the Pressure (Fig. 7)

- Attach a manometer to the hub of the needle (via three-way stopcock).
- Normal pressure ranges from 4.2 to 7.3 mm Hg
- Ensure the patient is relaxed and watch for good respiratory variation of the fluid level as the patient breathes normally.

- Check the CSF pressure.
- Remove the manometer.

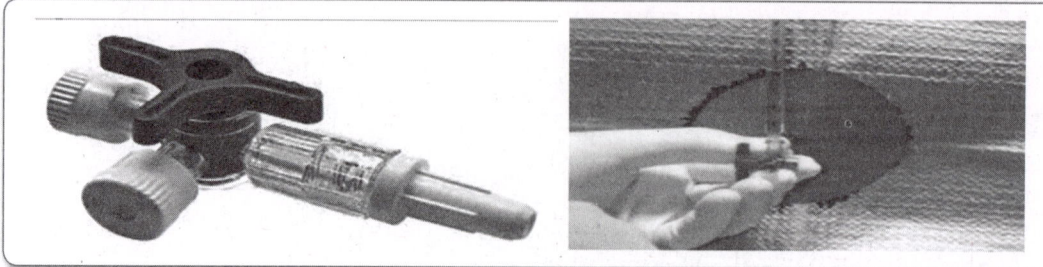

FIG. 7: Measuring opening pressure

Collect Cerebrospinal Fluid (CSF)

- Allow CSF to flow into sterile tube (Fig. 8).
- CSF can be collected for
  - Chemistry
  - Microbiology
  - Antibody testing (in particular Japanese Encephalitis IgM)
- Collect extra tube of CSF to hold in lab for possible later testing.

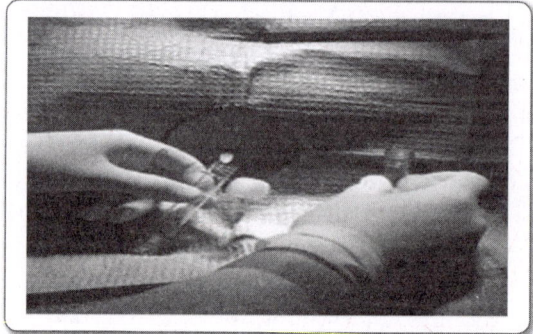

FIG. 8: Collecting CSF into sterile tubes

Final Steps

- Replace the stylet and withdraw the needle.
- Massage the puncture point with a sterile sponge.
- Cover with a Band-Aid.
  Advise adult patients to lie flat in bed for 3 hours and limit activity for 24 hours to minimize headache

Recording

- Label the tubes with the patient information and date of collection.
- Record the immediate results.

- ■ Appearance of CSF
  - ♦ Clear or turbid
- ■ Pressure of CSF

Documentation

Laboratory tests on CSF
- Cell count, differential
- Glucose
- Protein
- Gram stain
- India ink preparation
- Stain for acid-fast bacilli
- Viral, bacterial and fungal cultures
- Anti-JEV IgM ELISA
- JEV RT-PCR (If available)

Observation

Observe patient for next 24 hours
- Leakage of CSF
- Headache and backache
- Neurological observations
- Vital signs

TABLE 1: **Summary of typical CSF findings**

	Normal	Bacterial	Viral	TB
Cells	0–5 WBC/mm^3	>1,000/mm^3	<1,000/mm^3	25–500/mm^3
Polymorphs	0	Predominate	Early	± increased
Lymphocytes	5	Late	Predominate	Increased
Glucose	40–80 mg/dL	Decreased	Normal	Decreased
CSF plasma: Glucose ratio	66%	<40%	Normal	< 30%
Protein	50–40 mg/dL	Increased	± increased	Increased
Culture	Negative	Positive	Negative	+TB
Gram stain	Negative	Positive	Negative	Positive

LIVER BIOPSY

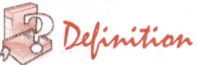 *Definition*

A liver biopsy is a quick, painless procedure designed to remove a sample of liver tissue for diagnostic purposes.

PRE-PREPARATION OF THE PROCEDURE

- Explain the procedure to parents

- Obtain a written consent
- Ensure the investigations
- Monitor the vital signs
- Administer sedative as prescribed
- Administer vitamin K

ARTICLES NEEDED

Before liver biopsy, a nurse prepares a biopsy kit which include
- Tru-cut needle or vim-silverman needle with the stylet or Menghini needle
- Procaine 1%
- Syringe with a needle
- Sterile cotton swab with antiseptic solution
- Sponge holder
- Kidney tray
- Tincture of benzoin
- Specimen bottles
- Pair of sterile gloves, gown and mask
- Center hole towel

PROCEDURE (FIG. 9)

- Explain the procedure.
- Give supine position.
- Palpate the liver and mark the best spot with a small red marker for inserting the needle.
- Clean the area on and around the biopsy mark with a Betadine solution.
- Place a sterile C shape sheet at the level of 10th intercostal space in the mid-maxillary line (right side).
- Administer a local anaesthetic (Lidocaine) by injection and makes a very small, deep incision at the biopsy mark.
- Insert a hollow biopsy needle into the liver through the incision.

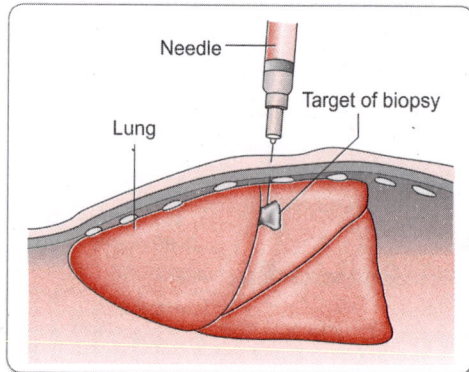

FIG. 9: Liver biopsy

- Quickly remove the needle immediately after collecting a sample of liver.
- Collect the sample into a jar of formalin.
- Keep the patient on a sideline position after putting a bandage over the wound.
- Send the biopsy to laboratory with proper documentation.

DURATION FOR A LIVER BIOPSY

From start to finish, the liver biopsy itself normally takes about 10 minutes. You will have to lie in bed for a few hours after it is over. However, during this time, your doctor will monitor you to make sure no internal bleeding or other complications occur. Outpatients usually leave the hospital after 4–6 hours.

INDICATIONS

- Indian childhood cirrhosis
- Hepatitis
- Unexplained hepatomegaly
- Tuberculosis (abdominal)

CONTRAINDICATIONS

- Prolonged prothrombin time
- Thrombocytopenia
- Blood dyscrasias
- Extrahepatic obstructive jaundice with enlarged bladder
- Cancer of the liver
- Infection of the lower lobe of the right lung

POSTPROCEDURE CARE

- Place a cotton pad over the site and turn the child on his right
- Keep a small pillow under his costal margin and make him stay in the same position
- Monitor vital signs every 10–15 minutes for first few hours and then every half an hour for first hours
- Watch for complications
- Send the specimen to the laboratory with the request form
- Keep the biopsy site aseptic

COMPLICATIONS

- Pneumothorax
- Injury to adjacent organs
- Hemorrhage
- Shock and collapse

RENAL BIOPSY

Renal biopsy is a specialized, minimally invasive procedure with some significant and serious but rare complications.

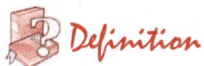 Definition

This is a medical procedure in which a small piece of tissue is removed from the kidney for microscopic examination.

INDICATIONS

- Steroid resistant nephrotic syndrome
- Severity of potential transplant rejection
- Condition with systemic lupus erythematoses
- For evaluation of response to the therapy and prognosis of the disease

CONTRAINDICATIONS

- Uncontrolled hypertension
- Severe anemia
- Bleeding diathesis
- Polycystic disease
- Solitary kidney
- Hydronephrosis
- Tumor of kidney or adrenal

ARTICLES NEEDED

- Tru-cut needle or vim-silverman needle with the stylette or Menghini needle
- Procaine 1%
- Syringe with a needle
- Sterile gauze pieces with antiseptic solution
- Sponge holder
- Kidney tray
- Tincture of benzoin
- Specimen bottles
- Pair of sterile gloves, gown and mask
- Center hole towel

SITE FOR BIOPSY

The usual site is 2 cm below and median to the tip of the 12th rib (lower border)

POSITION USED

Prone position with head turned to a side, arms abducted and forearms by the side of the head. A pillow is placed under his abdomen.

PREPROCEDURE PREPARATION

- Ensure that informed consent is gained and consent form is completed.
- Ensure that the child has a correctly labeled name band in place.
- Set baseline observation.
- Perform surgical hand scrub.
- Wear gloves.
- Paint the site with antiseptic solution.
- Infiltrate the site with 1% procaine injection.
- A 20 gauge long needle is inserted gradually in a sagittal plane parallel to the spine until it hits the kidney.
- The track is anaesthetized.
- Then needle with stylette is introduced along the anesthetized tract, while the patient takes deep breath, till it pierces the kidney capsule.
- The stylette is removed and the forked cutting needle is inserted to its full length.
- The child is asked to hold the breath and the other needle is pushed deeper so that it covers fully the forked needle.

- The whole apparatus is now rotated a full circle, leading to cutting of the biopsy material from the kidney.
- Then it is removed and the puncture site is sealed with tincture of benzoin.

POSTPROCEDURE CARE

- The child is kept in supine position and observed for 24 hours.
- He should be encouraged to take enough fluids and normal diet after he is out of the sedation.

COMPLICATIONS

- Microscopic hematuria; it is transparent and disappears in 2–3 days
- Pain abdomen
- Hematoma
- Intrarenal arteriovenous fistula
- Massive hematoma

BONE MARROW ASPIRATION

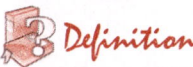 *Definition*

It is an invasive procedure by which a marrow is obtained through a fine bore needle.

INDICATIONS

- In case of aplastic anaemia and bone marrow suppression
- For diagnosis of malignant cells

SITE

- < 2 years:a point on the anterior-medial aspect of tibia about 2.5 cm below the tibial tubercle
- Older children—posterior or anterior iliac spine

POSITION

- If the posterior iliac crest is used, the child is positioned prone
- Anterior iliac crest supine position

ARTICLES NEEDED

A sterile tray containing
- Trocar and cannula of pediatric size
- 20 mL syringe
- Procaine 1%
- Syringe with a needle
- Sterile gauze pieces with antiseptic solution
- Pressure bandage

- Sponge holder
- Kidney tray
- Tincture of benzoin
- Specimen bottles/container/8–10 glass slides
- Pair of sterile gloves, gown and mask
- Center hole towel

PREPARATION OF CHILD AND PARENTS

- Explain the procedure
- Obtain a written consent
- Sedation should be given to the child to reduce the pain and anxiety.

PROCEDURE

- Perform surgical scrub
- Wear gloves
- Position the child appropriate to the site selected
- Paint the area with an antiseptic lotion
- Infiltrate the skin with procaine 1% up to the periosteum
- Place the center hole towel over the site
- Insert the trocar and cannula with rotating action through the skin down to the periosteum and then through the cortex into the marrow cavity
- As soon as the needle enters the cavity, some "give" is felt and there is sudden lack of resistance
- With the needle firmly fixed *in situ*, trocaris removed
- Fit a dry 20 mL syringe to the needle
- With strong suction for a few seconds, about 0.2 mL of marrow is aspirated into the syringe
- After aspiration, trocar is replaced and the needle is withdrawn
- The puncture site is pressed with a finger for 3–5 minutes
- A sterile dressing is applied over the site
- The aspirate is smeared in equal amounts on 8–10 glass slides which are waved in the air to accomplish fast drying

POSTPROCEDURE CARE

- Apply a small pressure bandage over the puncture site
- Send the specimens to the laboratory with the request form for diagnosis
- Document the procedure on nursing chart with date, time, site and procedure

NEEDLE BIOPSY

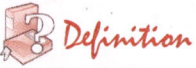 *Definition*

A needle biopsy (Fig. 10) is a procedure to obtain a sample of cells from the body for lab testing. The common needle biopsy procedures include fine needle aspiration and core needle biopsy. The needle biopsy may be used to take tissue or fluid samples from muscles, bones and organs, such as the liver or lungs.

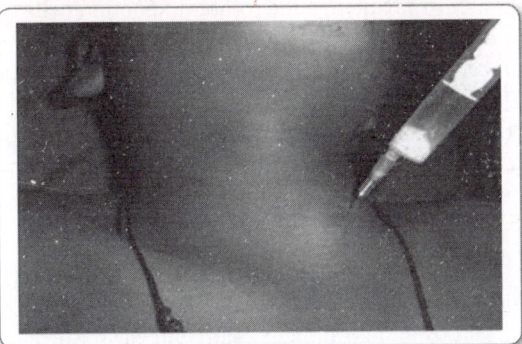

FIG. 10: Needle biopsy procedure

WHY IT IS DONE

The sample from your needle biopsy may help your doctor determine what's causing:

- A mass or lump—A needle biopsy may reveal whether a mass or lump is a cyst, an infection, a benign tumour or cancer.
- An infection—analysis from a needle biopsy can help doctors determine what germs are causing an infection so that the most effective medications can be used.
- Inflammation—A needle biopsy sample may reveal what's causing inflammation and what types of cells are involved.

RISKS

- Needle biopsy carries a small risk of bleeding and infection at the site where the needle was inserted. Some mild pain can be expected after needle biopsy though it is usually controlled with over-the-counter pain relievers or prescription medications.
- Fever
- Drainage from the biopsy site
- Swelling at the biopsy site
- Bleeding that does not stop with pressure or a bandage
- Pain at the biopsy site that worsens or is not helped by medication

PROCEDURE

- The skin above the area to be biopsied is swabbed with an antiseptic solution and draped with sterile surgical towels.
- The skin underlying fat and muscle may be numbed with a local anaesthetic although this is often not necessary with superficial masses.
- After locating the mass for biopsy using X-rays or palpation, a special needle of very fine diameter is passed into the mass.
- The needle may be inserted and withdrawn several times. There are many reasons for this:
  - One needle may be used as a guide, with the other needles placed along it to achieve a more precise position.

- Sometimes, several passes may be needed to obtain enough cells for the intricate tests which the cytopathologists perform.
- After the needles are placed into the mass, cells are withdrawn by aspiration with a syringe and spread on a glass slide. The patient's vital signs are taken again and the patient is removed to an observation area for about 3–5 hours.
- For biopsies in the breast, ultrasound-guided fine needle biopsy is the most common.

DURING NEEDLE BIOPSY

- First the interventional radiologist will use some form of imaging (CT, MRI, USG OR MAMMOGRAPHY) to determine the best site for the biopsy.
- Next a member of the interventional radiology team will wash the area where the biopsy will be performed and put local anaesthetic in the skin and deeper tissues to numb the area.

AFTER THE PROCEDURE

- After the biopsy, the patient may be asked to stay in the hospital for a brief times so that the staff can make sure you are all right.
- Most people go home between 1 and 4 hours after their biopsy.

COMPLICATIONS

- Very infrequent bleeding
- Infection.

18

Care of the Neonate

- ⊃ Immediate Newborn Care
- ⊃ Newborn Assessment
- ⊃ Neonatal Reflexes
- ⊃ Baby Bath

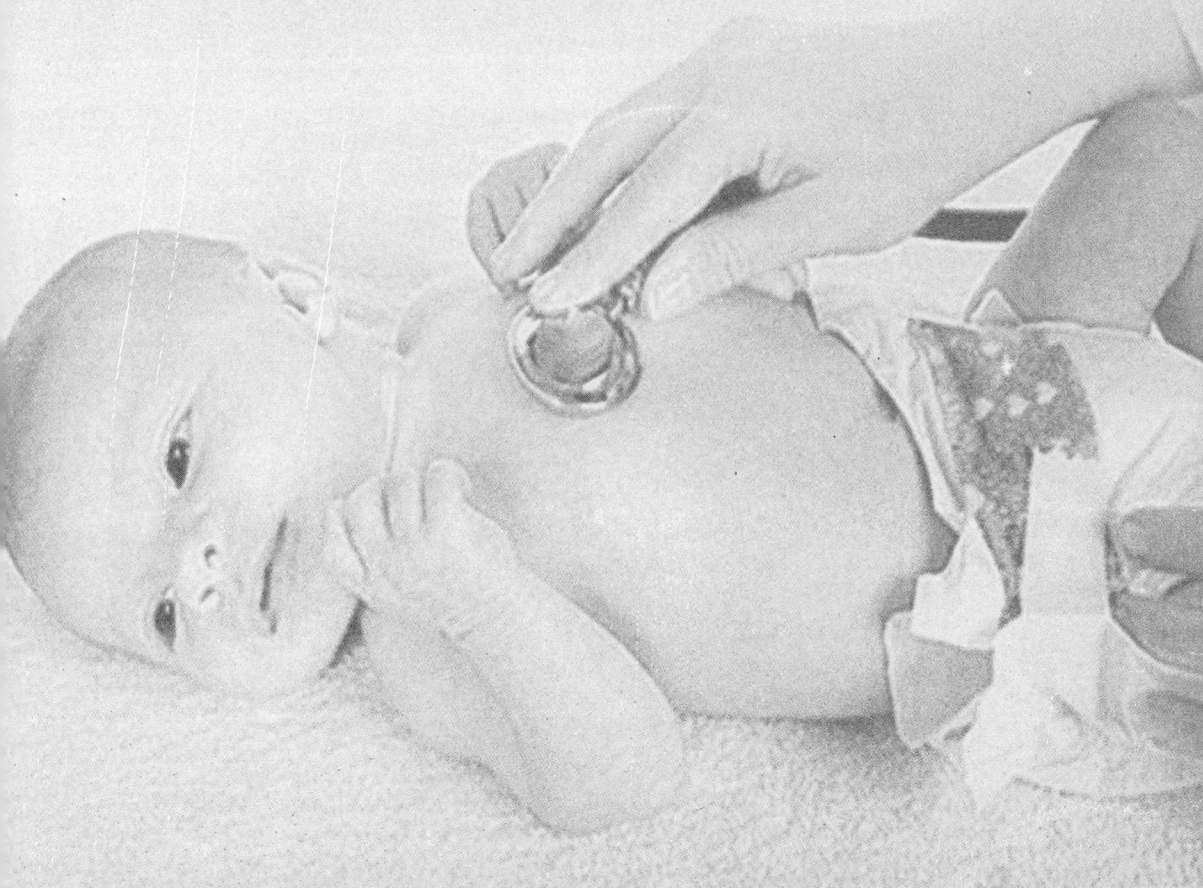

LEARNING OBJECTIVES

On the completion of this chapter, the pediatric nurse will be able to perform the following activities:
- Explain purposes of newborn care
- Explain immediate care of newborn
- Identify the problems of newborn
- Maintain routine care of newborn
- Enlist the equipment needed and the types of newborn assessment
- Prepare the child for assessment
- Identify abnormalities
- Develop skill in assessment of newborn from head to toe examination.
- Inculcate the skill in their practical field
- Explain the purpose of baby bath
- Develop skill in this procedure
- Inculcate the skill in their practical field
- Use of check list.

INTRODUCTION

The first 24 hours of life is a very significant and a highly vulnerable time due to critical transition from intrauterine to extrauterine life.

IMMEDIATE NEWBORN CARE

- **Airway**
- **Breathing**
- **Temperature**
- **Airway and breathing**
  - Suction gently and quickly using bulb syringe or suction catheter
  - Start in the mouth and then the nose to prevent aspiration
  - Stimulate crying by rubbing
  - Position properly—side lying/modified t-berg
  - Provide oxygen when necessary
- **Temperature**
  - Dry immediately
  - Place infant on warmer or use droplight
  - Wrap warmly
- **Apgar score—Standardized evaluation of the newborn**
  - Perform 1 minute and 5 minutes after birth
  - Involves five indicators:
    - Appearance
    - Pulse
    - Grimace
    - Activity
    - Respirations
- Anthropometric measurement

- Vitamin K administration
- Footprinting/marking
- Vital signs
- Dressing/wrapping
- Proper identification
- After delivery, gender should be determined
- Pertinent records should be completed including the ID bracelet
- Before transferring to nursery, ID tag should be applied.
- Do not remove vernix caseosa vigorously
- Cord care
- Weight/anthropometric measurements
- "Wrap in warm blanket
- Cover head with stockinet cap.

DAILY CARE

- Nutrition/feeding
- Elimination
- Weight
- Bathing and hygiene/grooming
- Obtain vital signs
- Rooming-in
- Note for any abnormalities.

NEWBORN ASSESSMENT

Assessment of the newborn is essential to ensure a successful transition from intrauterine to extrauterine life.

The types of newborn assessment are as follows:
- Immediate/initial newborn assessment
- Transitional assessment during period of reactivity
- Assessment of gestational age
- Physical examination
- Periodic assessment
- Prior to discharge

Purposes

To detect congenital anomalies and diagnose for early treatment

Articles Needed

A tray containing:
- Pair of gloves
- Tape measure
- Pneumatic otoscope with small head
- Ophthalmoscope

- Tongue blade
- Clear flexible ruler
- BP cuff pediatric size
- A bowel with sterile cotton balls
- Weighing machine
- Infantometer
- TPR tray
- A bright penlight with a pinpoint beam.

Principles of Examination

- Provision should be made to prevent neonatal heat loss during the physical assessment
- Examination should be done sequence wise
- Immediate/initial assessment at birth and within the first 4 hours after birth.

Apgar Scoring System

Apgar score

Criteria	0	1	2
Heart rate	Absent	Slow (<100)	>100
Respiratory effort	Absent	Slow, irregular	Good, crying
Muscle tone	Limp	Some flexion of extremities	Active motion
Reflex	No response	Grimace	Cough or sneeze
Color	Blue, pale	Body pink, extremities blue	Complete pink

Total score—10

The evaluation of all the five criteria should be made at 1 and 5 minutes after birth and are repeated at 5 minutes until the infant's condition stabilizes

> 0–3 score (severe distress)
> 4–6 score (moderate depression)
> 7–10 score (normal)

General Guidelines

- Keep the infant warm during examination
- Perform examination from general to specific
- One should start with least disturbance to the child
- Document all abnormal findings and provide nursing care.

General Appearance

- Posture
- Full term
- Symmetric
- Face turned to side
- Flexed extremities

- Hands tightly fisted with thumb covered by the fingers
- Special concerns:
  - Asymmetric
  - Fractured clavicle or humerus
  - Nerve injuries (Erb-Duchenne's Paralysis)
  - Breech presentation
  - Knees and legs straightened or in frog position.

Temperature

- **Site:** Axillary not rectal
- **Duration:** 3 minutes
- **Normal range:** 36.5–37.6°C
- Stabilizes within 8–12 h
- Monitor every 30 minutes until stable for 2 hours then every 8 hours.

Transitional Assessment (Period of Reactivity)

- **First period of reactivity:**
  Stage 1: During the first 30 minutes through which the baby is characterized as physiologically unstable, very alert, cries vigorously, may suck first greedily and appears very interested in the environment.
  Stage 2: It lasts for about 2–4 hours. Through this period, mucus production is decreased. The newborn is in the state of sleep and relatively calm.
- **Second period of reactivity:** It lasts for about 2–5 hours, through which the newborn is alert and responsive, heart and respiratory rate, gastric and respiratory secretions are increased and passage of meconium commonly occurs.
  Following this stage is a period of stabilization through which the baby becomes physiologically stable and a vacillating pattern of sleep and activity and passage of meconium commonly occurs.

General Examination

- **Posture:** In full-term babies, generalized flexion is seen. The neck and extremities are flexed. Pre-term babies may lie in frog-like posture.
- **Activity:** Normal neonates are alert and active. The baby may be irritable or drowsy if having any neurological problem.
- **Cry:** Normal neonate cries when hungry or wet. Weak cry is seen in pre-term or low-birth-weight babies.
- **Vital sign:** TPR are checked. The temperature of newborn ranges between 35.5°C and 37.5°C. Apical beat normally ranges from 120 beats/min to 140 beats/min. The respiratory rate ranges from 40 breaths/min to 60 breaths/min.
- **Temperature:** 97.5–99°F
- **Heart rate and rhythm measurement:** The heart rate of 120–160 bpm, blood pressure is only taken with the sign of illness.
- **Pulses (apical, femoral):** Strong and equal bilaterally.
- **Lungs (rate and rhythm):** The normal rate is 30–60 bpm. Period of apnea less than 15 second is normal.

Anthropometric Assessment

- **Weight:** The body weight of the neonate on an average is 2.5–3 kg. The neonate loses about 10% weight in first 10 days of life. Thereafter, baby gains about 25–30 g/day.
- **Length:** The average length of a neonate is 45–50 cm.
- **Head circumference:** Immediately after birth, moulding of skull may give inaccurate measurement of head circumference. So it should be measured after 48 h of birth. The normal head circumference is 33–35 cm. It may be larger in case of hydrocephalus and smaller in microcephaly or craniostenosis.
- **Chest circumference:** It is about 31–33 cm. It is 2–3 cm less than the head circumference.

Head-to-toe Examination

Head

- **Hair, color and amount:** Disturbed over top of head.
- **Circumference:** 33–35 cm.
- **Sutures and fontanels:** Sutures may override, called moulding, lasting 5–7 days; may bulge when infant is crying and coughing.
- **Anterior:** Diamond-shaped at front and top of head; closes between 12 and 18 months.
- **Posterior:** It is triangle-shaped at top, and to the back of the head, closes at birth or within 2 month.
- **Shape:** May be asymmetrical due to moulding, this should be disappeard in 5–7 days. May have edema formation or bleeding into subperiosteum.
- **Mouth/lips/gums:** The mouth should be round and symmetrical; hard palate should be intact with high arch.
- **Face:** The face may be asymmetrical due to soft tissue damage and swelling during birth process.
- **Palate:** Visualize the uvula and pharynx when the infant is crying. Tonsils are not visible in the newborn. Check for extrusion, sucking and rooting reflexes.
- **Eye:** Eye may be swollen and red from trauma of birth or from reaction to medication routinely used in the infant's eye upon admission. Tears may not be present for several weeks or even 3–4 months after that.
- **Ear:** The top of ear should be in level with outer canthus of eye. Ear cartilage should be formed so that ear holds shape.
- **Eyelid:** Edema
- **Nose:** The nose should be midline and symmetrical; check for nasal flaring. The nose may need to be suctioned with bulb. Syringe to maintain patency. Infants are obligate nose breathers they cannot breath through their mouth at birth.
- **Chest-circumference:** 31–33 cm; chest is almost circular. Slight intercostal retractions are normal.
- **Clavicles:** Check for bumps; clavicle may have been broken during birth. It should be smooth.
- **Breast:** The breast of the newborn of both the sexes may be swollen for the first few days due to level of maternal hormones. They may also excrete a whitish fluid that looks like milk.

Skin

- **Color, consistency, hydration:** The newborn baby is usually bright red with puffy skin. By the second to third day the color of the skin should be pink, dry and flaky. Normal color changes due to following conditions:
  - Acrocyanosis
  - Mottling

- **Jaundice:** Yellow skin due to accelerated breakdown of red blood cells
- **New born rash:** The eruption that appear 'hive like' and may appear and disappear at intervals during the first few days of life.
- **Birth Marks**
  - Mongolian spot
  - Stork bites
  - Vernix caseosa, lanugos'

Abdomen

- Bowel sounds: 2–4/min.
- Size contour: Usually rounded with prominent veins if scaphoid, suspect a diaphragmatic hernia; liver is usually palpable 2–3 cm below costal margin.

Vessels

- **Condition of cord:** The number of vessels will fall off in approximately 7–14 days. There may be brownish colored drainage after the cord falls off. Cord should be cleansed with alcohol and cotton balls until area is completely healed and drainage has ceased.

Extremities

- Arms/hands should have 10-finger look for polydactyly and sandactyly and the nail bed should be pink. Slight blueness is common when extremities are cold.
- **Legs/feet:** The sole of the toes should be usually flat with creases on anterior two-third of the foot; symmetry of legs with equal muscle tone and resistance to opposing flexion. Extremities usually have flexion; Ortolani's sign for hip dislocation.

Back/Spine

- **Spinal column:** Spine intact, no openings, masses or prominent curves. Spine usually rounded with none of curves seen later in life. Trunk in curvation reflex present. Stroke back along one side of the vertebral column will cause the infant to move hips towards the stimulated side.
- Posture/muscle tone
- Awake general appearance.

Urine

- Color and number of voiding.
- The urine should be voided within 24 hours with adequate hydration and should have 6–10 disperse per day.
- Urine is straw colored and odorless
- Dark yellow urine indicates dehydration.

Stools

- **Color:** Meconium is passed after 8–24 hours. After that infant begins eating; transitional stools are passed less sticky and brownish yellow. By the fourth day, a milk stool should be passed; breastfed infants have pasty yellow to golden stools with an odor similar to sour milk.
- **Placement of anus:** Midline
- **Patency of anus:** Patient anal opening parsing of meconium stool indicates patient anus.

NEONATAL REFLEXES

INTRODUCTION

- A reflex is an involuntary or automatic action that your body does in response to something without even having to think about it
- Neonatal reflexes—inborn reflexes present at birth and occur in a predictable fashion
- Normally developing newborn should respond to certain stimuli with these reflexes.

TYPES OF REFLEXES

General Body Reflexes

Moro Reflex/ Startle Reflex

- Begins at 28 weeks of gestation
- Initiated by any sudden movement of the neck
- Elicited by—pulling the baby halfway to sitting position from supine and suddenly let the head fall back
- Consists of rapid abduction and extension of arms with the opening of hands, tensing of the back muscles, flexion of the legs and crying
- Within moments, the arms come together again.

Clinical significance

- Its nature gives an indication of muscle tone
- Failure of the arms to move freely or the hands to open fully indicates hypotonia
- It fades rapidly and is not normally elicited after 6 months of age.

Palmar/Grasp Reflex

- Begins at 32 weeks of gestation
- Light touch of the palm produces reflex flexion of the fingers
- Most effective way—slide the stimulating object, such as a finger or pencil, across the palm from the lateral border
- Disappears at 3–4 months
- Replaced by voluntary grasp at 45 months.

Clinical significance

- Exceptionally strong grasp reflex—spastic form of cerebral palsy and kernicterus
- May be asymmetrical in hemiplegia and in cases of cerebral damage
- Persistence beyond 3–4 months indicate spastic form of palsy.

Plantar/Grasp Reflex

- Placing object or finger beneath the toes causes curling of toes around the object
- Present at 32 weeks of gestation
- Disappears at 9–12 months.

Clinical significance

- This reflex is referred to as the "readiness tester"
- Integrates at the same time that independent gait first becomes possible.

Walking/Stepping Reflex

- When sole of foot is pressed against the couch, baby tries to walk
- Legs prance up and down as if baby is walking or dancing
- Present at birth, disappears at approximately 2–4 months
- With daily practice of reflex, infants may walk alone at 10 months.

Clinical significance

- Premature infants will tend to walk in a toe-heel fashion while more mature infants will walk in a heel-toe pattern
- When the front of the leg below the knee or the arm below the elbow is brought into contact with the edge of a table, child lifts the limbs over the edge
- Present at birth, fades away rapidly in early months of life
- Reflex is readily demonstrable in the newborn and persistent failure to elicit it at this stage, is thought to indicate neurological abnormality.

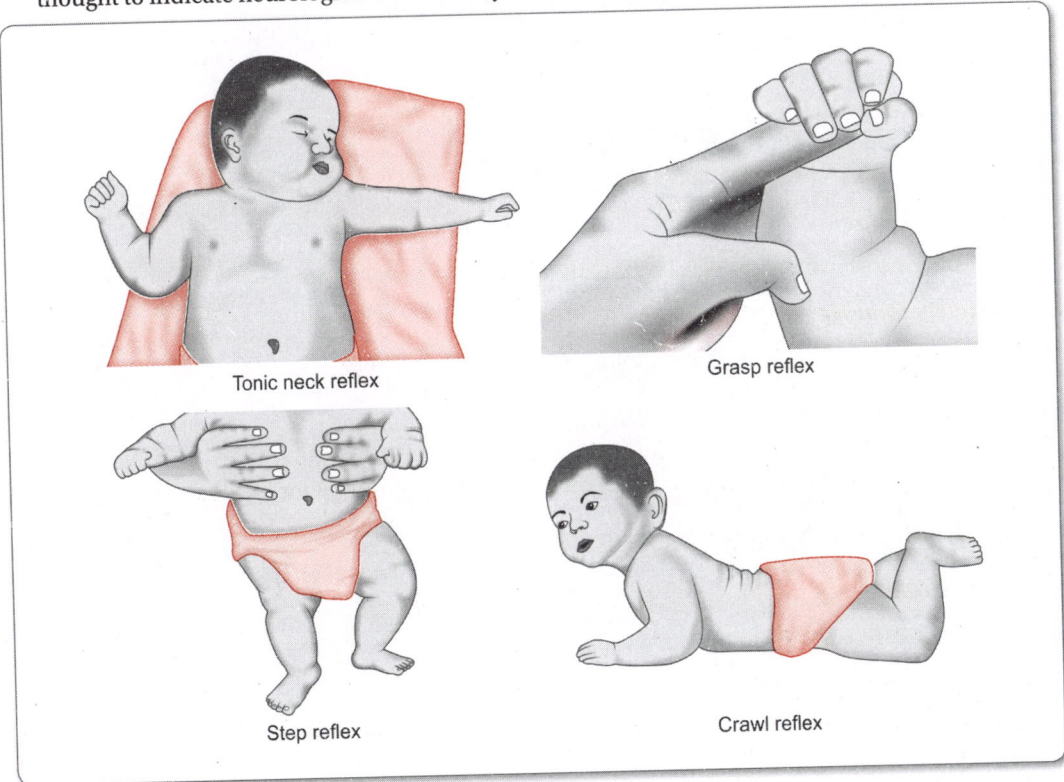

Tonic neck reflex

Grasp reflex

Step reflex

Crawl reflex

FIG. 1: Types of reflexes

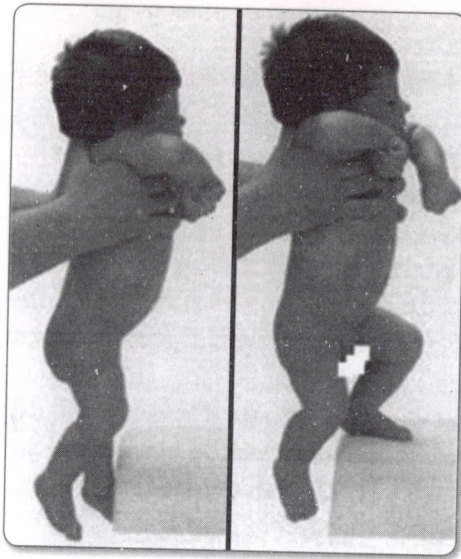

FIG. 2: Limb replacement reflex

Withdrawal Reflex

- Protective reflex
- **Stimulus:** A pinprick or a sharp painful stimulus to sole of foot
- **Response:** Flexion and withdrawal of stimulated leg
- Present at birth, persists throughout life.

Clinical significance

Absence of this is seen in neurologically impaired infants.

Asymmetric Tonic Neck Reflex

- Most evident between 2 and 3 months of age

Clinical significance

- The reflex fades rapidly and is not normally seen after 6 months of age
- Persistence is the most frequently observed abnormality of the infantile reflexes in infants with neurological lesions
- Greatly disrupts development.

Symmetric Tonic Neck Reflex

- To be present throughout life.

Clinical significance

- Examination is a part of some neurological extension of the head causes extension of the fore limbs and flexion of the hind limbs
- Evident between 2 and 3 months of age

- Not normally easily seen or elicited in normal infants
- May be seen in an exaggerated form in many children with cerebral palsy.

Babinski's Reflex

- Stimulus consists of a firm painful stroke along the lateral border of the sole from heel to toe
- Response consists of movement (flexion or extension) of the big toe and sometimes movement (fanning) of the other toes
- Present at birth, disappears at approximately 9–10 months
- Presence of reflex later may indicate disease.

Parachute Reflex

- Reflex appears at about 6–9 months and persists thereafter
- Elicited by holding the child in ventral suspension and suddenly lowering him to the couch
- Arms extend as a defensive reaction.

Clinical significance

- Absent or abnormal in children with cerebral palsy
- Would be asymmetrical in spastic hemiplegia.

Landau Reflex

- Seen in horizontal suspension with the head, legs and spine extended
- If the head is flexed, hip knees and elbows also flex
- Appears at approximately 3 months, disappears at 12–24 months

Clinical significance

Absence of reflex occurs in hypotonia, hypertonia or mental abnormality

Trunk Incurvation Reflex

- Stroking one side of spinal column while baby is on his abdomen causes
  - Crawling motion with legs
  - Lifting head from surface
- Present *in utero*, seen at approximately 3rd or 4th day
- Persists for 2–3 months

Blink Reflex

- A bright light suddenly shone into the eyes, a puff of air upon the sensitive cornea or a sudden loud noise will produce immediate blinking of the eyes
- Purpose—to protect the eyes from foreign bodies and bright light
- May be associated tensing of the neck muscles, turning of the head away from the stimulus, frowning and crying
- Reflexes are easily seen in the neonate and continue exams, particularly when evaluating coma
- Satisfactory demonstration of these reflexes indicate:
  - No cerebral depression
  - Contraction of appropriate muscles in response

Doll's Eye Reflex (Oculocephalic Reflex)

- Passive turning of the head of the newborn leaves the eye *"behind"*
- A distinct time lag occurs before the eyes move to a new position in keeping with the head position
- Disappears at within a week or two of birth
- Failure of this reflex to appear indicates a cerebral lesion.

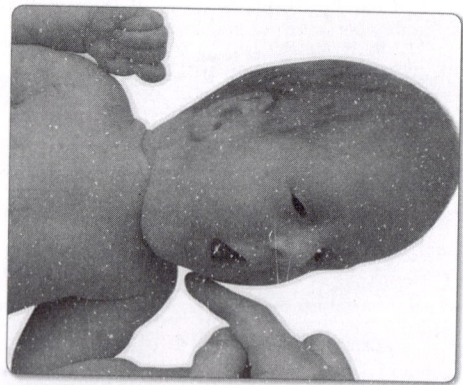

FIG. 3: Rooting reflex

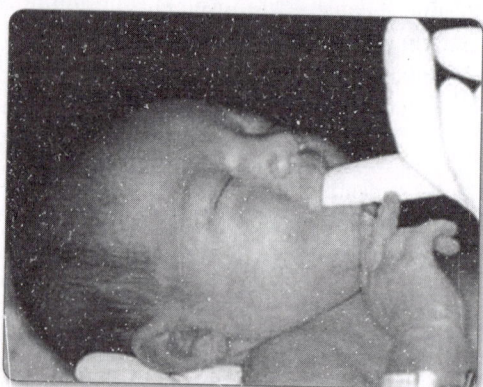

FIG. 4: Swallowing reflex

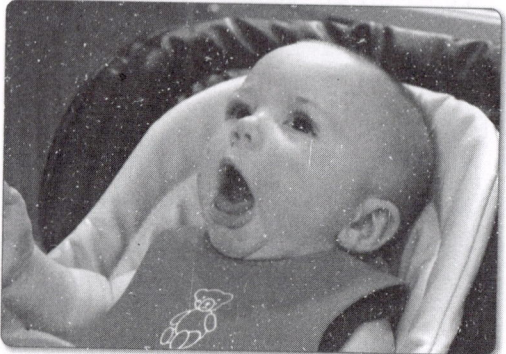

FIG. 5: Gag reflex

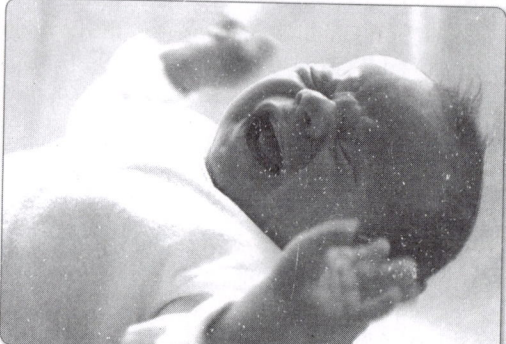

FIG. 6: Cry reflex

Oral Reflexes

Rooting Reflex

- Baby's cheek is stroked
- They respond by turning their head towards the stimulus
- They start sucking, thus allowing for breastfeeding
- When corner of mouth is touched, lower lip is lowered, tongue moves towards the point stimulated
- When finger slides away, head turns to follow it
- When center of lip is stimulated, lip elevates
- Onset—28 weeks IU
- Well established—32–34 weeks IU
- Disappears—3-4 months.

Clinical significance

- Persistence can interfere with sucking
- Absence of this is seen in neurologically impaired infants.

Sucking/Swallowing Reflex

- Touching lips or placing something in baby's mouth causes baby to draw liquid into mouth by creating vacuum with lips, cheeks and tongue
- Onset—28 weeks IU
- Well established—32–34 weeks IU.

Gag Reflex (Pharyngeal Reflex)

- Seen in 19 weeks of IU life
  - Reflex contraction of the back of the throat
  - Evoked by touching the roof of the mouth, the back of the tongue, the area around the tonsils and the back of the throat.

Functional significance

- It, along with reflexive pharyngeal swallowing, prevents something from entering the throat except as part of normal swallowing and helps prevent choking

Clinical significance

- Absence of the gag reflex—symptom of a number of severe medical conditions
- Damage to the glossopharyngeal nerve, the vagus nerve
- Brain death.

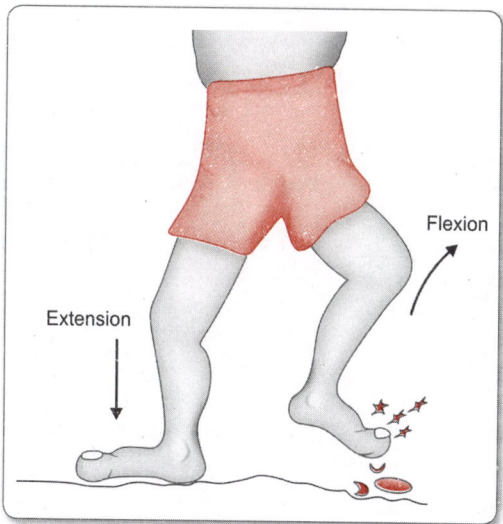

FIG. 7: Withdrawal reflex

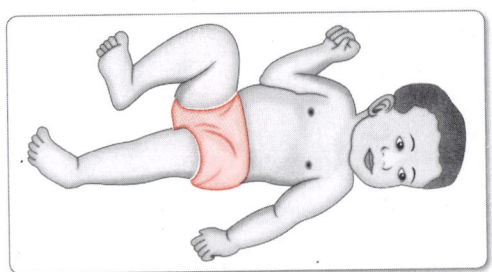

FIG. 8: Asymmetric tonic neck reflex

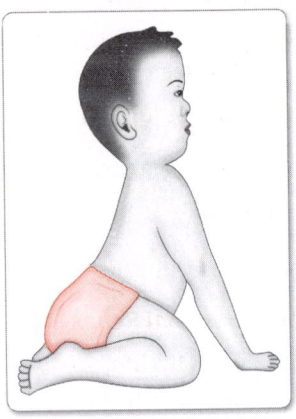

FIG. 9: Symmetric tonic neck reflex

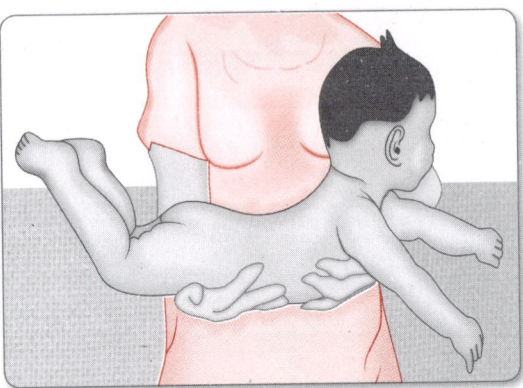

FIG. 10: Landaue reflex

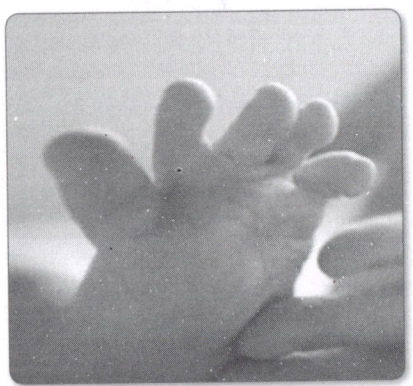

FIG. 11: Babiniskis's reflex

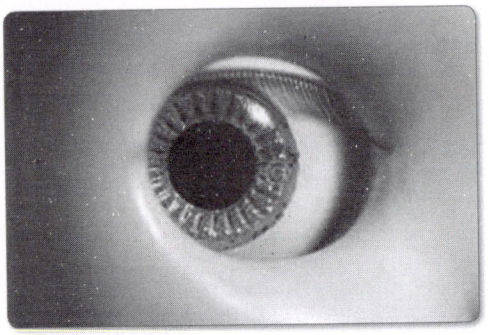

FIG. 12: Doll's eye reflex

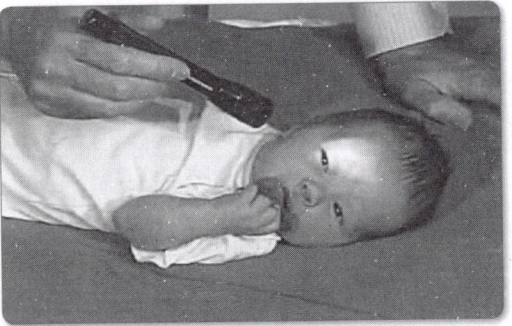

FIG. 13: Blink reflex

ESSENTIAL NEWBORN CARE PROCEDURE

- Call out the time of birth
- Deliver the baby on a warm clean towel on the mother's abdomen or chest
- Immediately dry the baby with a warm clean towel
- Remove the wet towel and wrap the baby in a warm dry towel
- Wipe both the eyes separately with sterile gauze from medial to lateral side
- Clamp and cut the umbilical cord in 1–3 minutes
- Place an identity label on the baby
- Leave the baby in between the mothers breast to initiate skin-to-skin care
- Cover the baby's head with a cap and cover the mother and baby with a warm cloth
- Encourage initiation of breast feeding.

EXAMINATION OF NEWBORN

Look at	Look for
Respiratory rate *The normal respiratory rate of a newborn baby is 30–60 breaths per minute with no chest indrawing or grunting on expiration*	• Respiratory rate consistently more than 60 or less than 30 breaths per minute • Grunting on expiration • Chest indrawing
	• Apnea (spontaneous cessation of breathing for more than 20 seconds)
Color *Babies born at term appear paler than preterm babies because their skin is thicker*	Palor
	Jaundice (yellow)
	Central cyanosis (blue tongue and lips; note that blue skin in addition to blue tongue and lips indicates a very serious problem)
Heart Rate (as determined using a stethoscope) *The normal heart rate of a newborn baby is 100–160 beats per minute, but it is not uncommon for the heart rate to be more than 160 beats per minute for short periods of time during the first few days of life, especially if the baby is distressed. If unsure of the heart rate, repeat the count*	• Heart rate consistently more than 160 or less than 100 beats per minute
Body temperature	• Less than 36.5°C
	• More than 37.5°C
Posture and movements (observed or history of) *The normal resting posture of a term newborn baby includes loosely clenched fists and flexed arms, hips, and knees. The limbs may be extended in small babies (less than 2.5 kg at birth or born before 37 weeks gestation*	• Opisthotonos (extreme hyperextension of the body, with the head and heels bent backward and the body arched forward)
	• Irregular, jerky movements of the body, limbs or face (convulsion or spasm)
	Jitteriness (rapid and repetitive movements that are caused by sudden handling of the baby or loud noises and can be stopped by cuddling, feeding, or flexing a limb)

Contd...

Look at	Look for
Muscle tone and level of alertness	• Lethargy (decreased level of consciousness from which the baby can be roused only with difficulty) • Floppiness (weak muscle tone; limbs fall loosely when picked up and released) • Irritability (abnormally sensitive to stimuli; cries frequently and excessively with little observable cause) • Drowsiness (sluggish) • Reduced activity
	Unconscious (profound sleep; unresponsive to stimuli and no reaction to painful procedures)
Limbs	• Abnormal position and movement of limbs • Baby's arms or legs move asymmetrically • Baby cries when a leg, arm or shoulder is touched or moved • Bone is displaced from its normal position
	Club foot (foot is twisted out of shape or position; e.g. heel is turned inwards or outwards from the midline of the leg) • Extra finger(s) or toe(s)
Skin *Some skin conditions are common and should not cause concern as long as the baby is otherwise normal.e.g. Milia, erythema toxicum*	• Redness or swelling of skin or soft tissues • Pustules or blisters
	• Blistering skin rash on palms and soles
	• Cut or abrasion
	• Bruise (bluish discoloration without a break in the skin, usually seen on the presenting part, e.g. buttocks in breech presentation)
	• Birth mark or skin tag (abnormal spot, mark or raised area of the skin)
	• Loss of elasticity
	• Thrush (bright red patches on skin in napkin area on buttocks, often scaly in appearance or with small white centers)
Umbilicus *The normal umbilicus is bluish-white in color on day 1. It then begins to dry and shrink and falls off after 7 to 10 days*	• Umbilicus is red, swollen, draining pus or foul smelling • Skin around umbilicus is red and hardened • Bleeding from umbilicus
Eyes	• Pus draining from eye • Red or swollen eyelids
	• Subconjunctival bleeding (bright red spot under the conjunctiva of one or both eyes)

Contd...

Look at	Look for
Head and face *The normal newborn baby's head may be moulded from a vertex birth; this will resolve spontaneously over a period of 3–4 weeks*	• Hydrocephalus (large head with bulging fontanel and widened sutures)
	Bulging anterior fontanelle
	• Sunken fontanelle
	• Unable to wrinkle forehead or close eye on one side; angle of mouth pulled to one side (facial paralysis) • Unable to breastfeed without dribbling milk
Mouth and Nose	• Cleft lip (split in lip) • Cleft palate (hole in upper palate connecting mouth and nasal passages)
	• Thrush (thick white patches on tongue or inside mouth)
	• Central cyanosis (blue tongue and lips)
	• Profuse nasal discharge ('snuffles')
	• Dry tongue and mucous membranes
Abdomen and Back	• Abdominal distension
	• Gastroschisis/omphalocele (defect of abdominal wall or umbilicus through which bowel or other abdominal organs may protrude)
	• Spina bifida/myelomeningocele (defect in back through which the meninges and/or spinal cord may protrude)
Weight	• Birth weight less than 2.5 kg
	• Birth weight more than 4.0 kg
	• Not gaining weight (proven or suspected)
Urine and stool *It is normal for a baby to have six to eight watery stools per day. Vaginal bleeding in the female newborn baby may occur for a few days during the first week of life and is not a sign of a problem.*	• Passes urine less than six times per day after day 2
	• Diarrhoea (increased frequency of loose stools as observed or reported by the mother; stool is watery or green, or contains mucus or blood)
	• The baby has not passed meconium within 24 h after birth

BABY BATH

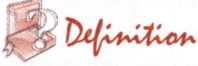 *Definition*

It is a procedure to clean the baby's skin by Luke-warm water.

PURPOSES

- To clean the baby's skin and increase skin integrity.

- To increase and maintain the proper blood circulation.
- To maintain the temperature at normal level.
- To make the bay refresh, till next bath.
- To prevent the baby from skin infections.
- To improve the skin functions and fragrance.

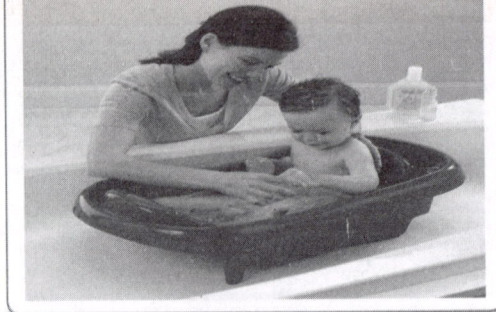

FIG. 14: Baby bath

ARTICLES NEEDED

- Mackintosh-1
- Large towel-4
- Small towel-1
- Nappy cloth
- Dress
- Soap in soap dish (Johnson and Johnson) Apron
- A clean tray containing
  - Sterile swabs for eye care and cord care in a bowl
  - Normal saline solution
  - Spirit in bottle
  - Bowl with cotton swabs
  - No absorbent cotton swabs
- Temperature tray
  - Bottle (3)-Disinfectant (2)
  - Clean water (1)
  - Clinical thermometer
  - Cotton swabs in bowl
  - Lignocaine jelly
  - Kidney tray
- Jugs (2)
- Bath basin (2)
- Bucket (2)

TYPE OF BABY BATH

Bath is of majorly four types:

- **Sponge bath:** This bath should be given to the infants who are acutely sick. It is given on the bed itself with the help of a soft sponge cloth. This bath is very commonly used for reducing the fever and maintaining the normal body temperature.
- **Tub bath:** Today in hospital settings, it is a common type of bath given to the baby. In this type of bath, the baby is submerged into the water in a bath tub or in a bath basin.
- **Lap bath:** In this bath, mothers of babies keep them on their lap and provide them bath. This type of bath is used when the tub bath is not possible. This bath is commonly used by mothers in rural areas.
- **Oil bath:** This type of bath involves application of oil, on the body which is applied all over the baby's body and then wiped off with cotton balls or with the rag pieces. This bath is used to remove

the vernix caseosa, when it fully covers the baby's body. This is applied for premature babies to maintain the body temperature because oil increases the body temperature.

Points to Remember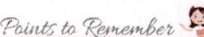

- Procedure should be explained to the mother before bath.
- Check the temperature of room, and if necessary, warm the room with the heater or blower.
- Keep the windows close and put off the fan to prevent the draughts.
- Adjust the position of the bath table to prevent from falling. Arrange the table against the wall.
- Keep the basin or tub bath on one side of the table and keep the baby's clothes on the other side, so that baby can be protected from fall.
- Place the mackintosh and towel over the table.
- Keep all the articles ready, nearby the table, before starting the procedure.
- Fill the warm water (100°F) in the bath tub, and the water should feel slightly warm to the inside of the wrist or elbow. Baby bath should be given before feeding. Make the baby calm before bath. Sometimes using powder on the skin of the baby may produce allergic rashes and reactions.
- Weigh the child before giving bath.

PROCEDURE

Preparation of the baby
- Check the physician's orders to see the specific precaution to be taken
- Assess the infant's need for bathing
- Check whether the child has taken feed in the previous one hour
- Check the articles available in the unit
- Check the body temperature
- Explain the procedure to the mother and let her be with the nurse

Preparation of the environment
- Close windows and put off fan to prevent draughts
- Adjust the position of the bath table
- Wash hands and wear apron
- Place the mackintosh and towel on the table
- Fill the basin half with warm water (37°C). The water should feel slightly warm to the inside of the wrist or elbow and should be kept over the table
- Bring the baby covered in a bath blanket to the table
- Wrap the baby in a big towel arranged on the table. Wrap in such a way that the hands are restrained in the towel
- Attend to infant's face, ears and scalp
- Wipe the eyes from inner canthus to the outer canthus using separate swab for each eye. Use one swab for one stroke. Observe for color of sclera, discharge, etc.
- With the wet hand, clean the face and back of the ears. Do not apply soap on the face. Dry the face by patting and not by rubbing
- Observe the mouth for thrush when the baby cries
- Use non-absorbent cotton to plug the ears or fold the ears over the external auditory meatus with thumb and index finger of one hand to prevent entry of water into the ears

- Pick up the baby securely by sliding hands until the baby's head is well supported by your palm. Hold the baby's head over the basin; wash the baby's head; apply soap and rinse well with water and dry the head thoroughly
- Discard the water and take fresh water
- Place the baby on the bath table unwrap the baby, wet the baby with wet hands. Apply soap all over the body, giving special attention to the neck, axilla, arms, finger, groin and toes
- Hold the baby firmly by supporting the head at the neck between the index finger and the other three fingers. Submerge gradually into the water in the tub to rinse the soap completely
- To pick up the baby, slide the hands under the baby's shoulders and grasp at the chest firmly. The head is supported by the fingers of both the hands. Make sure that your hands are free of soap.
- Take the baby from the water and dry him/her by patting gently; special attention is given to dry the body creases

Aftercare of the baby

- Thoroughly dry the baby with careful attention to the area around the cord stump if any
- Mummify the baby to prevent chill
- Comb the hair
- Handover the baby to the mother for feeding

Aftercare of articles

- Take the articles to the utility room. Disinfect the towels and the basin
- Clean and dry them and replace them in their proper place
- Wash hands

Recording

- Record the procedure in nurses, record with date, time, weight of the baby, temperature, observations and findings

Observation

- It is to be made for skin infection, oral thrush, cyanosis, jaundice, cord discharge, and respiratory changes

ACTIVITIES AFTER THE BATH

- Apply the baby oil, if indicated, and massage gently. Apply baby powder to increase fragrance, if indicated.
- Baby should be dressed with clean clothes.
- Comb the hair and wrap the baby in a blanket to prevent the chill.
- Give the baby to mother for feeding.
- Clean the articles and replace them. Disinfect the towels and bath basin.
- Do the handwashing.
- Do the recording and reporting of the procedure.

19

Emergency Care

➲ Neonatal Resuscitation
➲ Cardiopulmonary Resuscitation

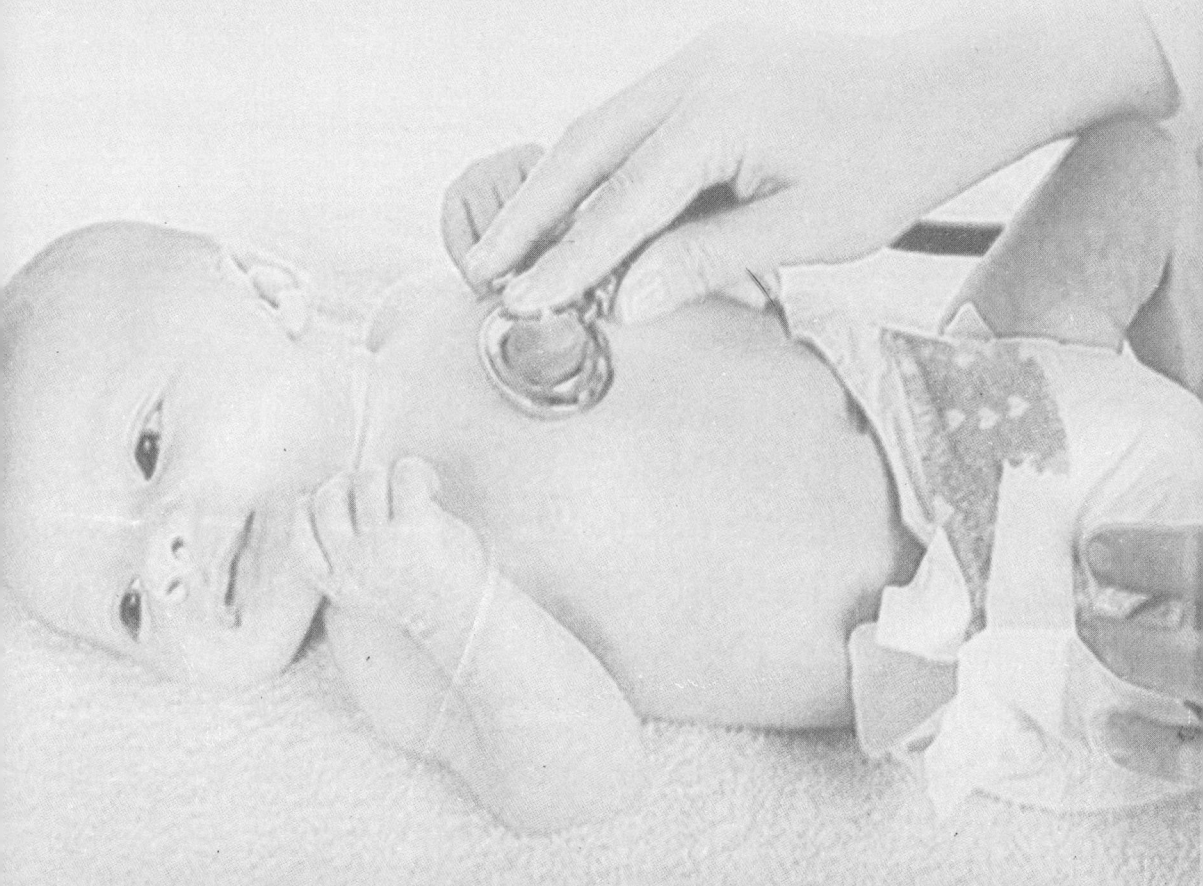

LEARNING OBJECTIVES

On the completion of this chapter, the pediatric nurse will be able to perform the following activities:
- Explain purpose
- Identify indications of neonatal resuscitation and CPR
- Enumerate the steps and methods of neonatal resuscitation and CPR
- Develop the skill in this procedure
- Inculcate the skill in their practical field.

NEONATAL RESUSCITATION

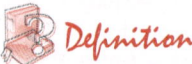 *Definition*

Neonatal resuscitation means to revive or restore life to a baby from the state of asphyxia.

Preparation for Birth

- Prepare personnels
- Test the function of equipment
- Test the function of bag and mask

Preparation in Delivery Room

Essential

- A draught free, warm room with temperature ≥25°C
- A clean, dry and warm delivery surface
- A radiant warmer/overhead lamp
- Two clean, warm towels/clothes
- A folded piece of cloth (1/2 to 1" thick)
- Infant masks in two sizes: size '1' for normal weight baby and '0' for small baby
- A suction device
- Oxygen (if available)
- A clock (with seconds hand)

Resuscitation of the Newborn Baby for 30 Seconds

- Deliver the baby on to the mother's abdomen
- Call the time of delivery
- Suction mouth and nose if the liquor is meconium-stained and baby not crying
- Use mucus trap for suction
- Suction mouth first, then nose ('m' before 'n').

T-ABC's of Resuscitation

Temperature

- Dry immediately
- Provide warmth

Airway

- Position
- Clear, if required

Breathing

- Stimulate

Circulation

- Assess heart rate
- Assess breathing of the baby

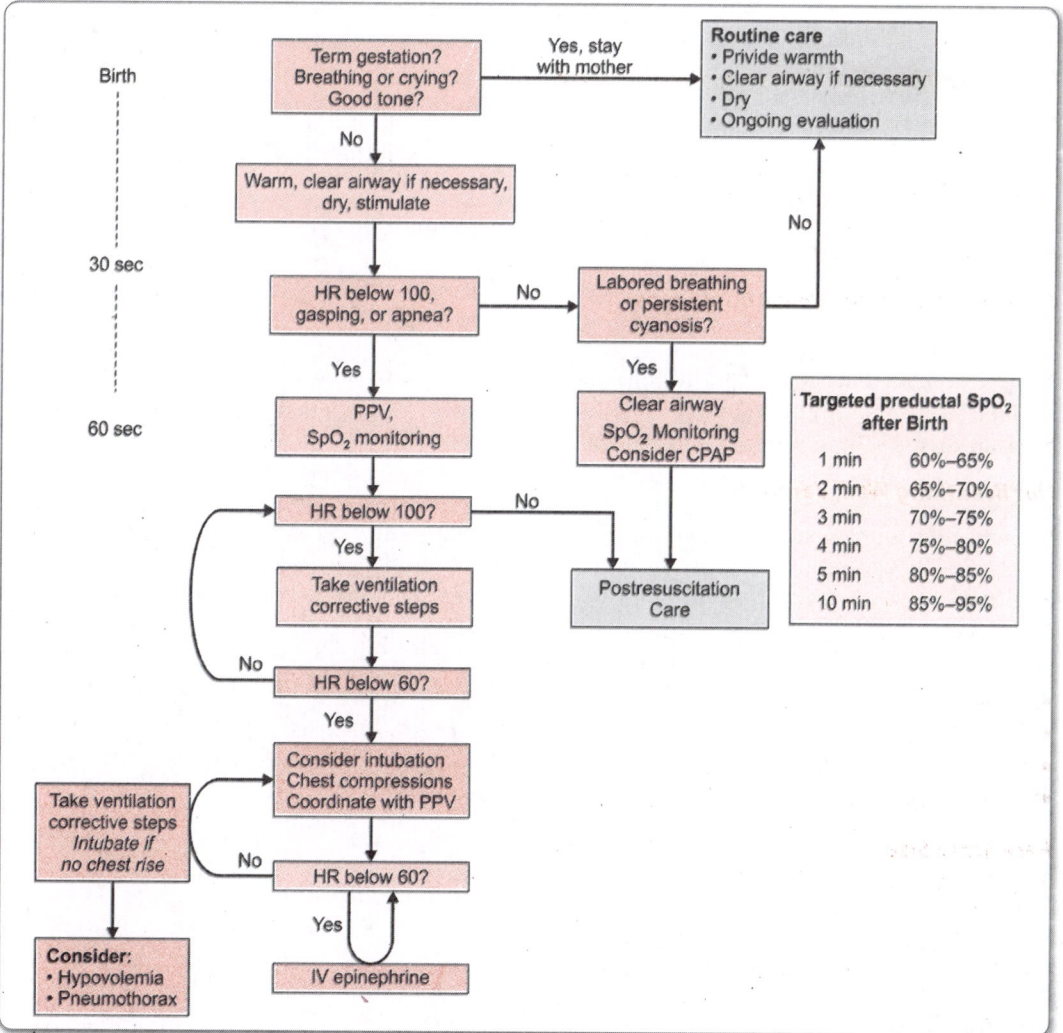

FIG. 1: Neonatal resuscitation

While Drying Assess Baby's Breathing

- Breathing well/crying routine care
- Not breathing well—initial steps

Initial Steps (For Babies not Crying)

- Cut the cord
- Place on the firm, flat surface
- Provide warmth
- Position the baby with neck slightly extended
- Suction the mouth, then the nose
- Stimulate, reposition

Baby Breathing Well or Crying: Routine Care

- Provide warmth
- Suction mouth and nose (if necessary)
- Cut cord in 1–3 minutes
- Keep the baby with the mother
- Initiate breastfeeding

Baby not Breathing Well: Initial Steps

- Tie and cut the cord.
- Tell the mother that her baby is having difficulty beginning to breathe and that you are going to help him. Tell her quickly but calmly.
- Transfer the baby to a warm clean, flat and dry surface.

Not Breathing Well: Ventilate

- If the baby is not breathing well then immediately ventilate the baby with bag and mask.

Positive Pressure Ventilation

Time: 30 seconds

Pressure is determined by four factors:

- Leak in the bag or equipment failure
- Any leaks between the mask and the face
- How hard the bag is squeezed (do not squeeze too hard; look for chest movement)
- Set point of pressure-release (pop-off) valve

Face Mask Size

Correct

It covers mouth, nose and chin but not the eyes.

Incorrect

Too large: It covers eyes and extends over chin.

Too small: It does not cover nose and mouth.

Face Mask Placement
- Correct position for assisted ventilation
- The mask usually is held on the face with the thumb, index and/or middle finger encircling the rim of the mask in shape of letter 'C'

Preparing for Positive-Pressure Ventilation
- Select correct-sized mask
- Position yourself at side or head of baby
- Position the head of the baby
- Clear airway

Effective Use of Bag
- Apply enough pressure to create noticeable, gentle rise and fall of the chest
- If baby appears to be taking a very deep breath, too much pressure is being used
- The primary sign of good ventilation is an increase in the heart rate

How to Squeeze the Bag?
Squeeze two to three times.

Look for Chest Movement
Reasons for inadequate or absent chest movements are as follows:
- The seal is inadequate
- The airway is blocked
- Not enough pressure is being applied

Points to Remember

Steps to Improve the Ventilation
- Reapply the mask and form a better seal
- Check the baby's position

If chest movement is inadequate or absent
- Clear the mouth and nose if necessary
- Try ventilating with the baby's mouth slightly open

If chest movement is inadequate or absent
- Increase the pressure to squeeze the bag harder

Success of ventilation improvement is indicated by
- Spontaneous breathing
  After taking steps to improve ventilation (if required), continue ventilation for 30 seconds and assess breathing and take appropriate decision

Assess Breathing

Breathing well
Regular breathing (40–60 per min)
- **Crying**
  - Not breathing well
- Gasping

Not breathing at all

Ventilate with the bag mask for 30 seconds and assess the area—breathing well observational care not breathing well

- Call for help
- Continue bag and mask ventilation
- Add oxygen, if available
  - Assess heart rate and feel the pulse at the base of umbilical cord or listen with the stethoscope
  - Count for 6 seconds and multiply by 10

Example: If you counted 13 pulsations in 6 seconds the baby's heart rate would be 13 × 10 = 130
Further action is based on evaluation of heart rate.

Assess heart rate

Heart rate normal 100 bpm or more. If heart rate is abnormal (less than 100 bpm) then continue ventilation.

Articles needed

- Suction equipment
- Bulb syringe
- Suction catheters with size number no 5, 6, 8 and 10 Fr
- 8 Fr feeding tube 20 mL syringe
- Meconium aspirator
- Face mask
- Oral airway
- Oxygen

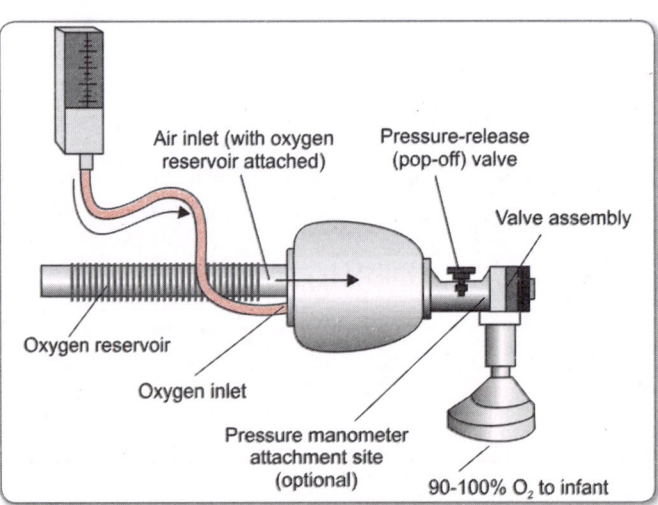

Air inlet (with oxygen reservoir attached)
Pressure-release (pop-off) valve
Valve assembly
Oxygen reservoir
Oxygen inlet
Pressure manometer attachment site (optional)
90–100% O$_2$ to infant

FIG. 2: Bag-mask equipment

- **Intubation Equipment**
  - Laryngoscopy—blade number 0 and 1
  - Battery for laryngoscope
  - ETT numbers 2.5, 3.0, 3.5 and 4.0 mm
  - Stylette scissor glove

- **Miscellaneous:** Radiant warmer, stethoscope, tape
- Syringe-needle, alcohol, umbilical catheter chest compression

Indications

If after 15–30 seconds of positive pressure ventilation with 100% F_1O_2 the heart rate is
- Below 60 bpm
- Between 60–80 bpm and not increasing

Technique

- One fingers breadth below nipple line, using two fingers
- One half to three fourth compression depth
- Accompanied by ventilations, ratio is 3:1

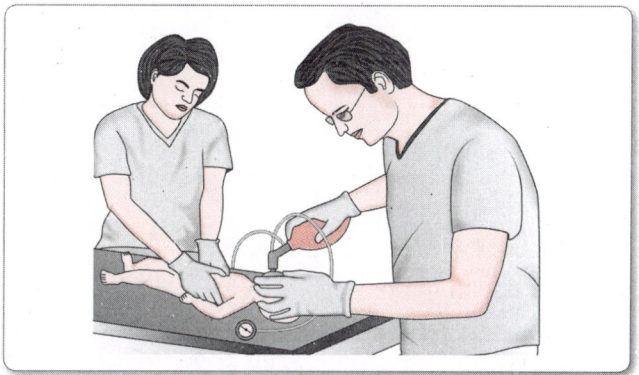

FIG. 3: Positioning the child for CPR

Principle

- Rhythmic compressions of sternum that
  - Compress the heart against the spine
  - Increases intrathoracic pressure
  - Circulate blood to vital organs
  - Chest compressions → compresses heart and increased intrathoracic pressure → blood pumped into arteries
- Pressure released → blood enters heart from veins

Positions

- Chest compressions are of little value unless the lungs are effectively ventilated
- Two persons are required
  - 1 – Chest compression provider should have access to the chest with his hands positioned correctly
  - 2 – Ventilation provider should be at head end to maintain effective mask–face seal or to stabilise ET tube.

Technique (Figs 4 and 5)

- **Thumb technique:** Two thumbs depress the sternum, hands encircle the torso and the fingers support the spine. This is the preferred technique for chest compression.

- **Two-finger technique:** Tips of the middle and index/ring finger of one hand compresses the sternum, the other hand supports the back
  Depth: One-third of the anteroposterior diameter of chest.
- Duration of downward stroke should be shorter than the duration of release
- Do not lift the fingers off the chest.

Points to Remember

Thumb Technique is Preferred because of:
- Better control of depth of compression
- Can provide pressure consistently
- Superior in generating peak systolic and coronary arterial perfusion pressure.

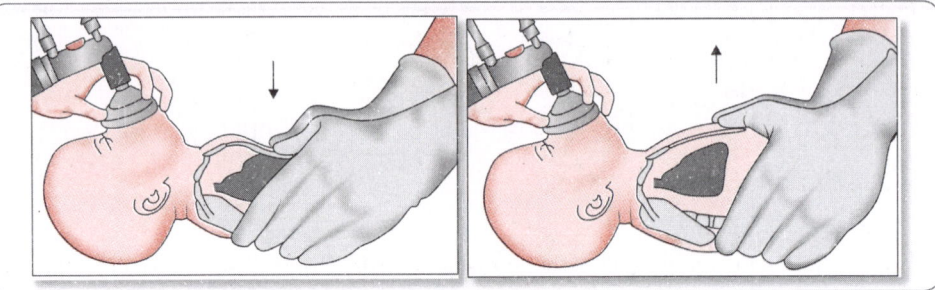

FIG. 4: Thumb technique

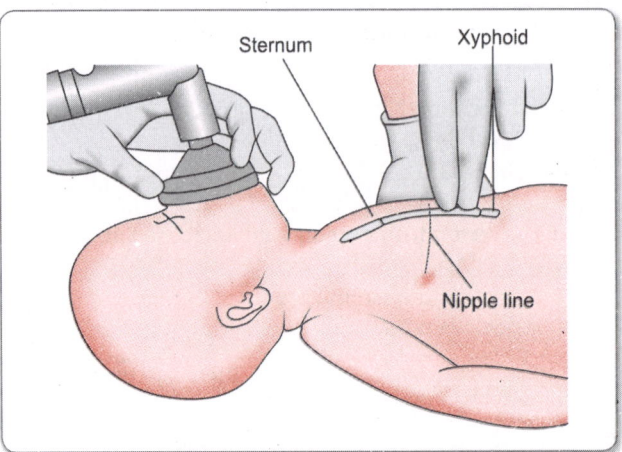

FIG. 5: Two finger

Procedure

- Look for meconium and suck mouth and nose at the mother's abdomen
- Dry the baby, remove the wet towel and wrap in the warm dry towel
- Assess breathing

- Cut the cord immediately
- Place the baby on a warm, firm flat surface
- Position the baby in slight neck extension using a shoulder roll
- Suction of mouth and nose
- Stimulate the baby
- Reposition and reassess breathing
- If not breathing provide bag and mask ventilation for 30 seconds, make sure that the chest rises
- Reasses the baby after 30 seconds of ventilation
- If still not breathing, continue bag and mask ventilation, start oxygen and assess the heart rate
- If the baby is still not breathing, continue bag and mask ventilation and refer to higher centre
- At any point if baby starts breathing, provide observational care.

Complications

- Laceration of liver
- Breakage of ribs

Medication

TABLE 1: Drug dosage

Drug	Preparation	Dosage	Rate/precautions
Epinephrine 1:10,000	1 mL	0.01–0.03 mg/kg 0.1–0.3 mL/kg	Give rapidly IV or ET Repeat every 3–5 min (ET: dilute to 1–2 mL with NS)
Volume expanders -NS orRL -5% ALBUMIN -O-VE BLOOD	40 mL	10 mL/kg	Give IV over 5–10 min
Naloxone 0.4 mg/mL 1.0 mg/mL	1 mL 1 mL	0.1 mg/kg 0.2 mL/kg 0.1 mL/kg	Give rapidly IV or ET preferred
Reserved for prolonged resuscitation only			
Sodium bicarbonate (0.5 mEq/mL = 4.2% solution Dopamine (6 × weight in kg = mg of dopamine diluted to 100 mL)	20 mL 10 mL × 2 100 mL	2 mEq/kg (4 mL/kg)	Give slowly over at least 2 min, IV only infant must be ventilated; continuous infusion by pump

- **Indication**
  - HR < 80 bpm despite 100% O_2 and chest compression 30 sec
  - No heart rate

Care after procedure

- Continuously observe the child for at least 48–72 hours
- Check the color of the skin and assess the respiration
- Check the temperature every hourly
- Start IV infusion to maintain the fluid level

- Provide oxygen if needed
- Check the head and jaw positions because tongue may fall back and can obstruct the airway
- Discard the waste materials.

Post resuscitation care

- Provide warmth
- Observe breathing, temperature, color and CFT
- Monitor blood sugar
- Watch for complications*; refer, if so
- Initiate breastfeeding, if well

Follow-up Care after Successful Resuscitation

For the Baby

- The mother and the baby should be kept together in skin-to-skin contact.
- Encourage the mother to breastfeed her baby as soon as it is ready.
- Assess the baby's attachment at the breast. Help the mother breastfeed if needed.
- Record what has happened in the baby's notes and in the labour record.

For the Mother and the Family

- After resuscitation, explain to the mother and the family what has happened and how the baby is now.
- Keep the mother and baby in the delivery room and do not separate them.
- Never leave the woman and the newborn alone. Monitor them every 15 minutes during the first hour.

CARDIOPULMONARY RESUSCITATION (CPR)

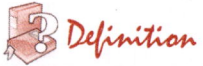 Definition

Cardiopulmonary resuscitation is a pediatric emergency procedure which is used to revive the child when breathing is stopped due to respiratory or cardiac arrest.

Mechanism of Cardiac and Respiratory Failure

The cardiovascular and respiratory systems depend on each other. In our body, the heart needs more oxygen than any other organ, because it works regularly and beats to pump the blood in the body. When the lungs stop working, the heart fail occurs. Similarly when heart stops, after sometime ventilation of lungs also fails. It occurs due to the lack of oxygen transported by the cardiovascular system to the respiratory centre which is situated in the medulla oblongata. The cardio-respiratory failure can be identified by the sudden fall in the arterial oxygen tension and increase in the arterial carbon dioxide content. The signs and symptoms of cardiac arrest are apnoea, absence of carotid and femoral pulse, dilated pupils, cyanosis, unconsciousness and fits, etc.

Indications of CPR

- **Cardiac arrest:** In children, various causes which leads to cardiac arrest such as to myocardial infarction, hypotension, drowning, electric shock, drug reactions, pulmonary embolism, hypothermia, hemorrhage, carbon monoxide and other types of poisoning and electrolyte disorders.

- **Respiratory arrest:** In children, it can occur due to drowning, foreign body, airway obstruction, drug toxicity, suffocation, injury, etc.

Points to Remember

General Instructions for Nurses
- Nurses should have good skill in CPR techniques.
- CPR should be given when the circulation of blood and respiration suddenly stopped.
- There is no use of CPR techniques in children during the last stage of incurable illness, and when respiration, heart beat have been absent for more than 6 minutes.
- Nurse should recognize the signs of cardiac arrest and start immediate artificial ventilation of the lungs with external cardiac compressions.
- CPR should be started within 3–4 min in order to prevent permanent brain damage.
- CPR should not be discontinued for more than 5 seconds till the normal circulation and ventilation are started.
- The cardiac compression and ventilation ratio should be 5:1, it means five cardiac compression and one ventilation (respiration). The rate of cardiac compression depends on the age group of child.
- Nurse should observe the complications carefully, for example, damage to spinal cord, fracture of ribs, gastric distension, pneumothorax, rupture of liver, etc.
- Stop the CPR when circulation and respiration are established. Nurse can stop CPR by observing the constriction of pupils, by feeling the pulse, by blood pressure, improvement in skin color and rhythmic movement of respiration.
- Nurse should observe the vital signs regularly till 24–48 hours to prevent another attack.

Articles Needed

For CPR, no equipment are necessary for performing the procedure because it needs good physical skill to perform the activities as early as possible, but for the saving of time and effective emergency care following articles should be available in any intensive care unit 24 hourly.

- Ambu bag and mask.
- Oxygen administration sets—tubes, mask, humidifier, etc.
- IV infusion set for emergency medications.
- Laryngoscope according to the age of children.
- Endotracheal tubes for different sizes.
- Oropharyngeal and nasal airways.
- Set of tracheostomy.
- Defibrillator and cardiac monitors.
- Suctions apparatus.
- Gauze pieces in a container for cleaning the mouth or wiping the lips.
- Some emergency drugs such as sodium bicarbonate, epinephrine, cardiac and respiratory stimulant drugs, etc.

Preparation of Child

- Do not waste time by explaining the procedure to the child and the family members.
- Make the surrounding area free from crowd and room should be well ventilated; arrange adequate space for the rescuers to work.
- Place the child on a hard surface or a hardboard should be placed under the child's thorax region.

- Remove the clothings from child's chest and make it free to observe the child's heartbeat and respiration. Remove the tight clothings from the child's neck.
- Place the child on his back without any pillow, hyperextend the head and neck.
- Start the procedure within the immediate time (about 4–6 min after the cardiac arrest).

Procedure

The CPR should be started in the following phases.
- A—Airway clearance.
- B—Breathing maintenance by artificial ventilation.
- C—Circulation maintenance.
  First clear the airway then breathing should be assisted, and last circulation should be established. When two nurses are available then breathing and circulation can be started simultaneously.

Airway Clearence

Airway can be obstructed by the some foreign matter, for example, secretions, vomitus, etc. the airway clearance can be completed by following the maneuvers techniques.

- **Head tilt–chin lift maneuver:** In this technique, the nurse should place one hand on the child's forehead and give the firm backward pressure with the palm to tilt the head back, while fingers of the other hand should be placed under the bony part of the lower jaw near the chin and lift up to bring the jaw forward.
- **Jaw thrust maneuver:** In this techniques, hold the angles of the patient's lower jaw and lift with both the hands, one hand should be on one side and on other hand should be on another side; keep the mandible in forward direction.
- **Back blow and chest thrust :** It is used commonly for the infant and below 1-year age children. In this method, place the infant on the forearm and keep face downward; rest this arm on the same side thigh of the nurse. The jaw of the infant should be supported by the hand. Now give five forceful back blows between the infant's shoulder blades with the heel of your hands. Now turn the infant immediately and position the infant face up on your forearm; arm should rest on the thigh; head should be lowered in position; give four chest thrust on about the centre of the breastbone. In this, infant technique is sandwiched between the hands of the nurse.
- **Heimlich maneuver techniques:** This technique is used for the conscious or unconscious child who have age above 1 year. This technique can be given to the child in both standing and lying positions.
- **Child with standing position:** In this technique, the child will be in standing position, and the nurse should stand behind the child. Make a fist with one hand, place the thumb side of the fist against the child's abdomen, at the midline, just above the navel and well below the xiphoid process. Grasp your fist with your other hand, give quick upward thrusts. Repeat the procedure about 5–10 times or repeat the procedure until the object is expelled or until the patient's consciousness improve.
- **Child with lying position:** In this technique, the nurse should stand or kneel at the child's feet as appropriate. Place the heel of one hand on the child's abdomen in midline just above the navel and below the xiphoid process. Keep the other hand on the top of the fist. Give the upward and midline thrust.

CPR Cardiopulmonary Resuscitation (Fig. 6)

1. Attempt to wake the child and call for help.

2. Begin chest compression

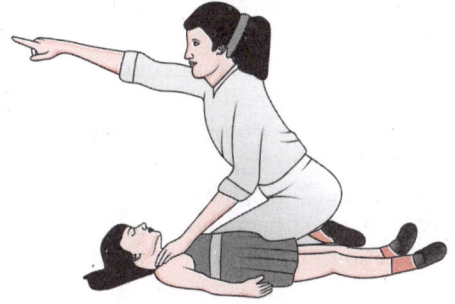

3. Open the airway

4. Begin rescue breaths.

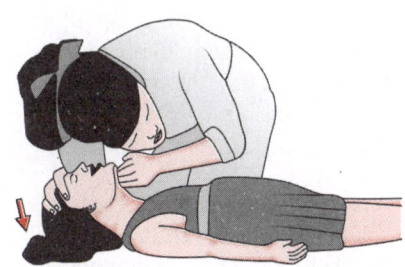

5. Repeat chest compressions.

6. Repeat rescue breaths.

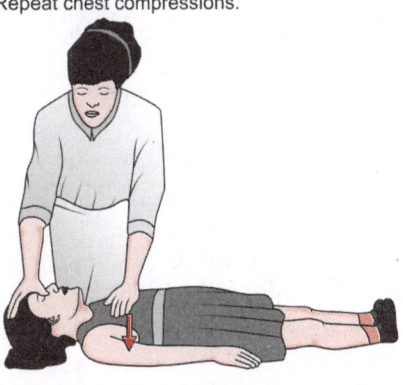
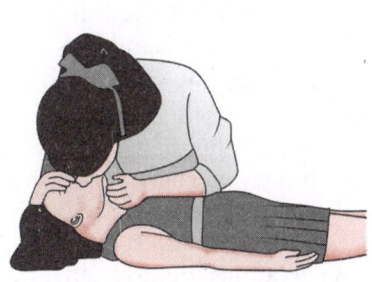

FIG. 6: Giving CPR to child

Initiate Breathing

After airway clearance, breathing should be initiated immediately. It can be improved by mouth to mouth breathing.

- **Mouth-to-mouth breathing:** Place the child in supine position. Tilt back the head, lift the chin, pinch the child's nostrils close, by using an index finger and the thumb of the hand near the child's face. Take deep breath, place your widely opened mouth over the child's mouth and nose and blow enough to make the chest rise; observe the chest expansion. If air does not go in, retilt head and breathe again. For infants and small children, both the mouth and nose should be covered by the nurses mouth; for infants, the nurse should use only puffs of air from the cheeks for sufficient insufflations. For older children, only the mouth is covered and the nostrils are firmly pinched to make air tight. Nurse should use small breath of air to inflate the child's lungs. The nurse should not have any type of respiratory tract infections. After each inflation, take your mouth away from the child's mouth. In children, inflation rate of about 20–30 times per minute should follow. When cardiac compressions are given to the child then compression and ventilation ratio should be about 5:1; it means for every five cardiac compression there should be one ventilation.
- **Bag and Mask ventilation:** In this method, an instrument known as Ambu bag is used, this Ambu bag is connected with the mask. This mask should be placed on child in such a position that it should cover the mouth as well as nose of the baby. On each five cardiac compressions, one ventilation by the Ambu bag should be given. This Ambu bag should deliver 100% oxygen and should not have a pressure relief valve. In this method, the child should be positioned on back with the chin forward and the neck slightly extended. Placing a rolled towel under the shoulders can help in maintaining this position. The mask is placed over the child's nose and mouth with a tight seal; now bag is rhythmically compressed. Observe the child for chest expansion.

Maintain Circulation

Maintenance of circulation can be achieved by external cardiac compression. The cardiac compression should be started with ventilation. Five cardiac compressions and one ventilation should follow.

External cardiac compression is compression of heart in the mediastinum between the sternum and vertebral column. In this technique, the child should be placed in supine position on a firm surface. For the firm surface, we can use a hardboard, a table or any other hard clean surface. In this method, heart is compressed between the sternum and the vertebrae.

Techniques of cardiac compression

It depends on the age of the child

- **External cardiac compression for infants:** For infants, the nurse should draw an imaginary line between the nipples and place the index finger farthest from the head of the infant under the intermammary line at the point where it intersects with the sternum bone. Now locate the area at one finger width below this intersection, other method—locate the area at the middle and ring finger width below this in section. Now by using tips of index and middle finger, chest is compressed to a depth of 0.5–1 inch at the rate of 100 times per minutes.
- **External cardiac compression for the young children (1–8 years):**
  - The compression for the child between 1–8 years of age are applied to the lower half of the sternum.
  - Compression should be applied by heel of one hand.

- Chest is compressed to a depth of 1–1.5 inches at the rate of 80–100 times per minute.
- Other one hand should be on forehead.
- **External cardiac compression for the older children (above 8 years of age):**
  - If child is above 8 years of age, the adult method is used for cardiac compression.
  - The heel of one hand is placed on the lower third of the sternum above the xephoid process (2 inches above the xephoid).
  - Place the heel of the other hand on the top of the first hand.
  - Keep the fingers elevated from the chest wall or they may be interlocked.
  - Compress the mid-sternum about 1–2 inches depth at the rate of about 60–80 compression per minute.
  - Assess the vital signs of child and compression must be followed until the patient starts spontaneous respiration and pulse.

Care after Procedure

- Continuously observe the child for at least 48–72 h.
- Check the color of skin the and assess the respiration.
- Check the temperature every hourly.
- Start IV infusion to maintain the fluid level.
- Watch for convulsions which may occur due to brain damage or acidosis.
- Insert endotracheal tube to maintain an open airway for the unconscious patients.
- Provide oxygen if needed.
- Check the head and jaw positions because tongue may fall back and can obstruct the airway.
- Discard the waste materials.
- Do the proper recording and reporting of procedure.

Complications

During CPR, following complications may occur
- Gastric distension may occur due to air.
- Damage to the spinal cord at cervical region due to hyperextension of the head and neck.
- Fracture of ribs, sternum and collarbone occur.
- Pneumothorax can occur.
- Intra-abdominal hemorrhage.
- Rupture of liver, myocardium and stomach can occur.

20

Restraints

- ➲ Purposes
- ➲ Articles Needed
- ➲ Types of Restraints
- ➲ Complication/Hazards of Restraints

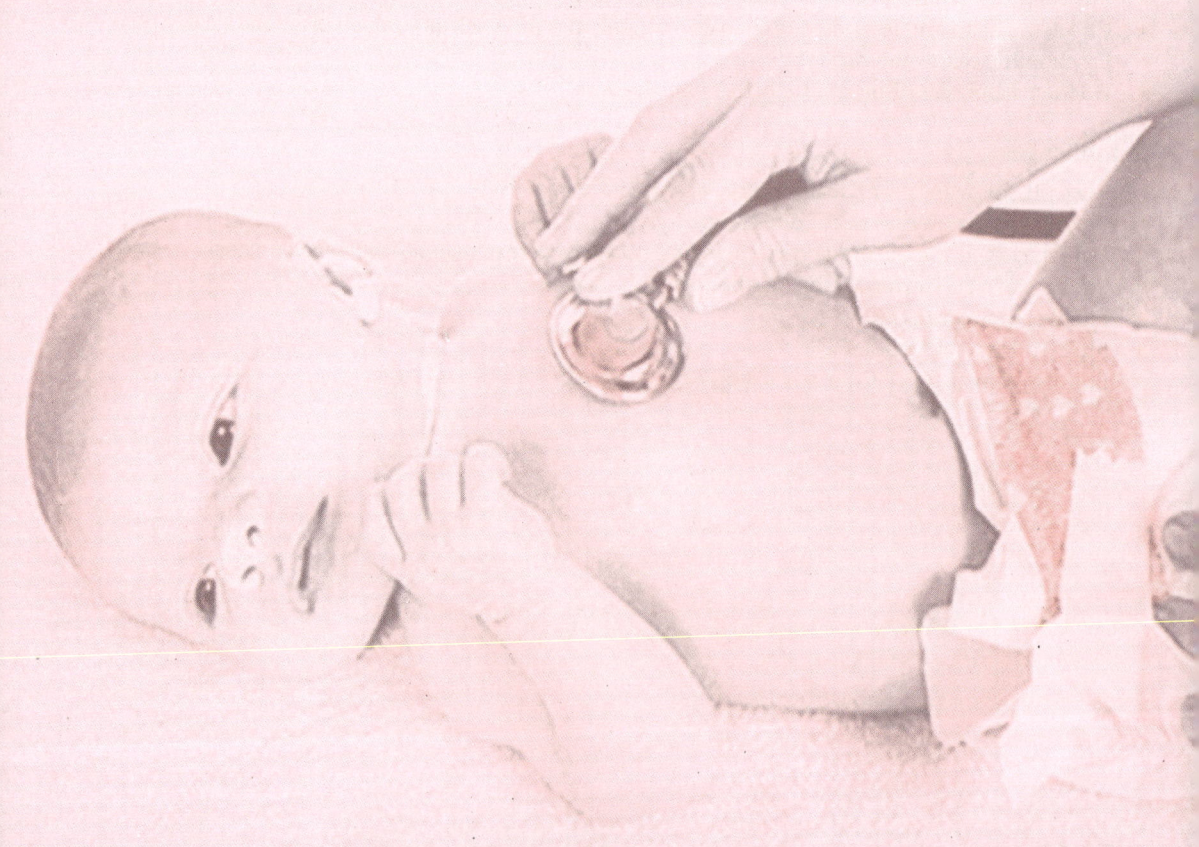

LEARNING OBJECTIVES

On the completion of this chapter, the pediatric nurse will be able to perform the following activities:
- Explain purposes and different types of restraints
- Develop skills in restraints procedures
- Inculcate these skills in their practical field

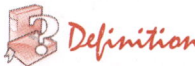 *Definition*

Restraints are protective and mechanical devices which are used to minimize the movements and protect the child from injury. These restraints are made up of linen, canvas, leather, plastic, metal or wood.

PURPOSES

- To carry out the physical examination
- To provide the safety to child
- To complete the diagnostic and therapeutic procedures
- To protect the child from injury
- To maintain the child in prescribed position
- To reduce the discomfort of the child during some tests and procedures such as specimen collections.

ARTICLES NEEDED

- Baby blanket or draw sheet
- 4" bandage for clove hitch knot
- Cotton pads
- Restraint cloth with pocket
- Wooden or plastic strips (spatula) to keep in pocket for elbow restraint
- Scissors to cut the bandage
- Jacket for jacket restraint
- Adhesive tape to fix the bandages

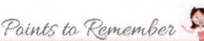 *Points to Remember*

- Always select a safe and appropriate restraint.
- Restraint should not be too tight and it should not interfere with the normal circulation.
- Use appropriate cotton pads for maintaining the comfort of the child.
- Restraint should demonstrate to the child, on the child's doll, to gain the cooperation and reduce the anxiety.
- Explain the restraint, and it is important that the child should be able to understand.
- Always maintain comfort to the child and maintain body alignment.
- Open the restraint knot when the side rails are raised to prevent traction.
- Observe the restraint every 20–30 minutes to prevent any complications.
- Change the side of the child to prevent pressure sore.
- Do not lie too tightly. If should be easily releasable.
- Do not provide purposeless restraining.
- Recording and report the observations properly.

TYPES OF RESTRAINTS

- Mummy restraint
- Elbow and knee restraint
- Abdominal restraint
- Extremity restraint (clove hitch knot)
- Finger restraint
- Crib-net restraint
- Jacket restraint
- Safety belt restraint
- Side rails.

Mummy Restraint

Mummy restraint is used for the children to restrict the movement of limbs. It is used for examination, procedure and treatment of head, neck and face, for example, scalp venipuncture, ear examination, eye irrigation, gastric gavage and gastric lavage.

For mummy restraint, take a blanket or draw a sheet and spread it over the bed or table. Place the baby on backside. Keep one hand of the baby near the body and wrap the baby's body by holding the corner of sheet and tuck it under the body in the opposite side. Now place another hand near the body and wrap the child's body by holding another corner of sheet and tuck it. Now, take the rounded sheet at bottom near the leg and fold it towards the chest and tuck it at upper level of sheet or we can pin it at the lower level of sheet. It restricts all the extremities.

Modified Mummy Restraint

In modified mummy restraint, we expose the chest and abdomen and limbs are restrained. This method is used to examine the chest and abdomen together.

Elbow and Knee Restraint

Elbow and knee restraint is used to control the flexion of elbow and knee. In this method, a readymade cloth with 6–10 pockets is used. Place the cotton on sides of elbow and knee and keep the wooden or plastic strips in pockets of cloth. These pockets are vertical. Place the cloth on elbow and knee and adjust it with central location and tie the both side strips properly.

The elbow restraint is used in case of face and head surgeries. Cleft lip and cleft palate, scalp vein infusion, heat injuries and sutures are good examples of using the elbow restraint.

Abdominal Restraint

This restraint is used to hold the infant in a supine position on the bed. Abdominal restraint should not be too tight, so that it cannot interfere with respiration and bowel movement. For this restraint, use wide size wooden strips. Place the cotton pad appropriately to provide the proper comfort.

Extremity Restraint (Ankle and Wrist)

This involves the extremity (one or more) restraint to complete some procedures. It is used to immobilize the extremities. There are various methods used for ankle and wrist restraint, for examples.

Clove Hitch Knot Restraint (Fig. 1)

It is used to immobilize the leg or arm. The material for clove hitch can be soft cloth, crepe bandage and 2-inch wide gauze bandage. First apply the cotton pad over the wrist and ankle to provide comfort. Prepare a figure of eight by the bandage and place it in the wrist or the ankle. Tie the bandage by knot. The knot should not be too tight or too loose. The child can remove the knot if it is too loose too tight knot can interfere in blood circulation. The fingers and toes should be checked for discoloration or any skin rash, etc.

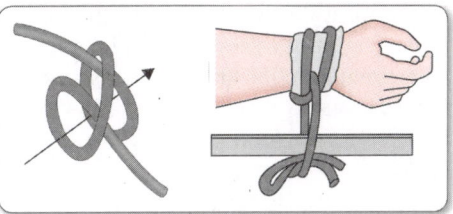

FIG. 1: Clove hitch knot restraint

Finger Restraint (Fig. 2)

It can be completed by making a mitten. The mitten covers the all fingers of a hand and restricts the movement of fingers. The hand can be wrapped by the gauze or hand can be put in a bag like pouch and tie it properly at the wrist of the child. Finger restraint is used in case of facial surgeries, burns, intravenous infusion, any eczema of face and body parts. Keep the mitten soft and it should not interfere with circulation.

Crib-Net Restraint

In this method, a net is used to cover the child's cot. Net is attached to the cot frame. This net restraint is used to prevent the children from climbing over the side rails of cot.

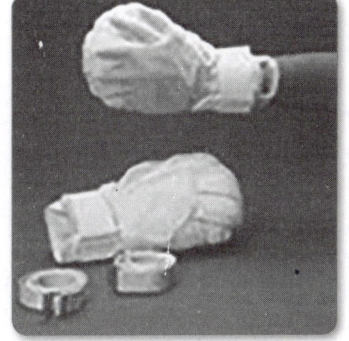

FIG. 2: Finger restraint

In this net, when side rails are up, the child can stand but cannot climb over the side rails of cot. Inside the crib net, the child is totally free to move and no movement is restricted. It mainly prevents the child to climb and fall from the side rails of cot.

Jacket Restraint

In this method, a jacket made up of soft cloth and leather is used. This jacket have laces at the back and two long strips. The laces are tied at back, and long strips are tied at the sided below the rails under the mattress. The child can sit and sleep in supine position while wearing the jacket. It can be used on chair also. This restraint is used to avoid the child from climbing over the side rails, climbing out from chair, bed, cot etc. It prevents the child from fall and injury. Some other types e.g. chest restraints are also used for children who are sitting on a chair or wheelchair to maintain their position and to prevent them from fall and injury.

Safety Belts

These are made up of electrically non-conductive materials. These belts are used on stretcher and operation tables to prevent the children from falling. These belts go around the childs waist and tied to the frame of bed under the mattress.

Side Rails

These are available especially in children cot. The rails are made up of iron or steel. These can be raised whenever need arises and can be decreased, as per convenience. The main pupose of side rails are to prevent from fall and can be used for other restraints. These are used for children with convulsive disorders also.

Splints

These are prepared devices which are used to restraint the movements of extremities. These are made up of plastic, card board, hard paper, cotton and gauze pieces. These can be applied where-ever needed.

Other Restraints

These are plaster cast, sand bags, bandages, binders, slings, etc. and used to restrict the movements of different parts of the body.

COMPLICATION/HAZARDS OF RESTRAINTS

If restraint is not used properly, it can cause various complications or hazards.
- It can interfere the child's muscular development due to lack of movement.
- If restraint is too tight, it causes obstruction in blood circulation, tissue damage, redness, scar formation, discoloration of the skin etc.
- Dislocation of the shoulder joint may occur if the child struggles during application of arm restraints.
- Development of the pressure sore, if the child is kept restricted for longer period of time and does not have frequent change of position and skin care.
- Hypostatic pneumonia due to immobility.
- Ischemia or nerve damage due to constrictive restraints.
- Psychic injury to the child, the child feels that he/she is punished, alteration in self body image.
- Disturbance in psychosocial development.
- To avoid these hazards, the caregiver or nurse should follow the safety precautions.
  - Use proper amount of cotton pads and do not use too tight restraint.
  - Always follow continuous observation on the child. In case of any complication, release the restraint and consult the doctor.
  - Maintain proper recording and reporting.

21

Elimination Needs

➲ Urinary Catheterization
➲ Suprapubic Catheterization

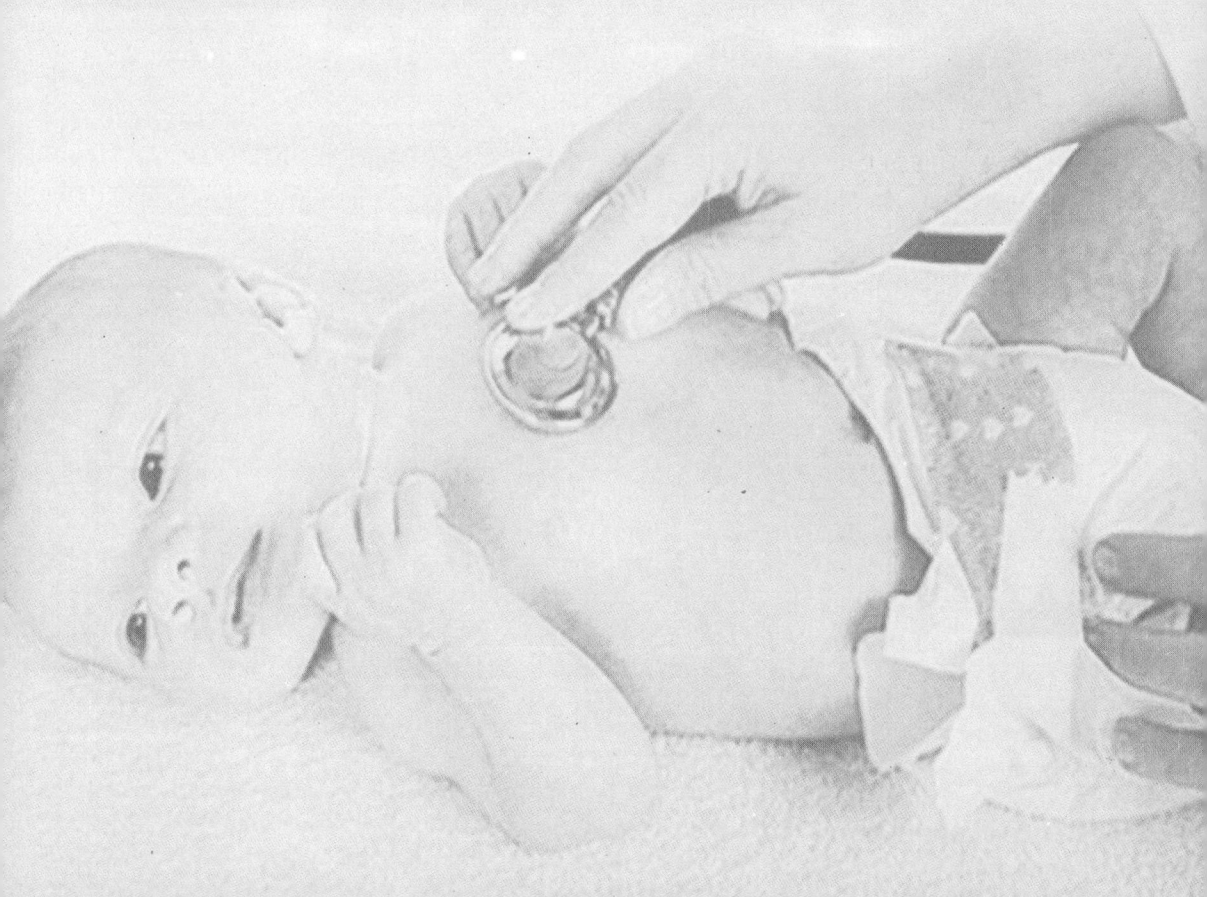

LEARNING OBJECTIVES

On the completion of this chapter, the pediatric nurse will be able to perform the following activities:
- Explain the techniques and purpose of urinary catheterization
- Explain the techniques and purpose of suprapubic catheterization

URINARY CATHETERIZATION

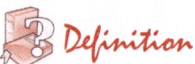 **Definition**

Urinary catheterization is the insertion of the catheter through the urethra into the bladder for withdrawal of urine.

INDICATIONS

- To relieve urinary retention
- To obtain a urine specimen
- To measure residual urine
- Management of child with spinal cord injury
- For diagnostic testing such as voiding cystourethrography or urodynamics
- Surgical procedures involving pelvic or abdominal surgery
- Post surgery and critically ill patients to monitor urinary output
- Refractory bladder outlet obstruction
- Prolonged bladder with urinary retention

ARTICLES NEEDED

- A sterile tray containing
- Disposable sterile gloves
- Drapes: One fenestrated, one non-fenestrated
- Lubricant
- Cotton balls with container
- Two artery forceps
- 10 mL syringe with sterile water to inflate the balloon
- Sterile catheter
- Appropriate type and size
- Sterile water
- Adhesive tape
- Urinary drainage bag with tubing
- Catheter selection for specimen

Size of catheter according to the age slot

0–1 year	4–5 Fr. feeding tube
1–2 years	4–5 Fr. feeding tube
12–18 years	8 Fr. feeding tube

Selecting Indwelling Catheter

Size of catheter according to the age slot

0–1 year	5 French feeding tube
1–2 years	6–8 Fr. Foley's catheter
12-18 years	8–14 French. Foley's catheter
15–18 years	Fr. Foley's catheter for boys

PROCEDURE

- Gather appropriate equipment and place these into a sterile field
- Perform hand hygiene
- Wear sterile gloves

For Female Child

- Place a sterile drape under buttocks.
- Gently separate and pull up the labia minora to visualize the meatus by using nondominant hand and hold the labia open throughout the procedure.
- Swab the meatus from the proximal to distal end using sterile povidone iodine dipped swabs.
- Lubricate the catheter and insert into the urethra until urine is obtained.
- Advance the catheter to an additional 2.5–5 cm
- Inflate the balloon with sterile water
- Connect the Foley's catheter to closed drainage system
- Clean the meatus and labia with providone and wipe it with wet swab
- Praise the child for cooperation

For Male Child

- Grasp the penis with non dominant hand and retract the foreskin and it should remain through-out the procedure.
- Place the sterile drape under the penis.
- Using the sterile cotton swab, clean the glans and meatus with providone iodine.
- Hold the penile shaft just under the glans to prevent the foreskin from contaminating the area.
- Lubricate and insert the catheter while gently streching the penis and lifting it to 90° angle to the body.
- Ask the child to inhale deeply and advance the catheter at that time.
- Once urine is obtained, advance the catheter to the hub.
- For intermittent catheter, insert only up to recommended length.
- Inflate the baloon with sterile water.
- Connect the Foley's catheter to closed drainage system.
- Clean the glans and meatus with water and wipe it with wet swab.
- Replace the retracted foreskin.
- Secure the catheter to either child's abdomen or thigh.
- Praise the child for cooperation.

Instillation of Lidnocaine Gel

Infant	0.5–1.5 mL
Toddler	1.5–2.5 mL
School age	2.5–5 mL
Adolescent	3–5 mL

SUPRAPUBIC CATHETERIZATION

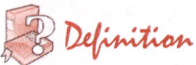 Definition

It is basically an indwelling catheter that is placed directly through the abdomen. The catheter is inserted above the pubic bone; this catheter must be placed by an urologist.

INDICATIONS

- Chronic infection of the urethra or periurethral glands
- Long-term catherization
- Urethral stricture
- Urethral trauma
- Urine analysis
- Phimosis

ARTICLES NEEDED

- Sterile gloves
- Antiseptic solution
- Gauze pieces
- Sterile drapes
- Anesthetic solutions without epinephrine
- Syringe 10 mL
- Needles 18 and 25 gauge
- Syringe 60 mL
- Percutaneous suprapubic catheter set
- Needle obturator
- Connecting tube
- One-way stop cock
- Sterile urine leg bag
- Drain sponges
- Skin tape or nylon suture 3.0 with a needle driver

PATIENT PREPARATION

- Explain the procedure
- Take a written consent

PROCEDURE

- Perform hand hygiene and wear gloves
- Administer analgesics
- Clean the lower abdomen
- Shave the suprapubic area
- Palpate the distended bladder and mark the insertion site at the midline and 2 inches above the symphysis pubis
- Apply an antiseptic solution from the pubis to the umbilicus
- Apply sterile drapes and verify the insertion site by palpating anatomical land mark
- Fill the 10 mL syringe with the local anesthetic agent and use the gauge needle to raise a skin at the insertion site
- Advance the needle through the skin and using the 11 no. blade, make a 4 mm stab incision at the insertion site with the blade facing inferiorly
- Insert the needle obturator into the Malecot catheter and lock it into the part by twisting it so that the needle tip projects 2–5 mm from the distal end of the catheter
- Connect the 60 mL syringe to the part of the needle obturator
- Place the tip of the catheter
- The practitioner's hand should be placed on the lower abdominal wall and the unit should be stabilised between the thumb and index finger
- The dominant hand should be used to advance the unit while aspirating until urine enters the syringe
- Once urine enters the syringe, advance the unit 3–4 additional centimeters into the bladder
- While securing the unit with the nondominant hand unscrew the obturator from the catheter and then completely withdraw the obturator needle
- Connect the extension tubing to the catheter and connect the tubing to a urinometer or a leg bag
- Gently withdraw the catheter to lodge the wings against the bladder wall
- Undrape the patient and apply the skin preparatory solution to drain dressing around the catheter at the insertion site
- Stitch the catheter to the skin

POST-PROCEDURE CARE

- Monitor the child for obstruction diuresis for 2–3 hours
- The inserted site should be inspected and cleaned with soap and water to prevent cellulitis and abscess formation
- Simple irrigation with normal saline should resolve most of the catheter obstructions
- Ensure that the child drink fluids adequately
- Ensure that drainage bag is below the level of waist.

NURSE'S RESPONSIBILITY

- Monitor vital signs, intake and output and fluid status
- Encourage coughing and deep breathing exercises and early ambulation
- Ensure adequate drainage and tube patency
- Irrigate the catheter as ordered
- Observe the skin around the insertion site for signs of infection and encrustation
- When changing a suprapubic catheter, speed is very important; the new catheter should be inserted within 5–10 minutes of removal of the old catheter

22

Pre- and Postoperative Nursing Care of a Child

➲ Preoperative Care
➲ Postoperative Care

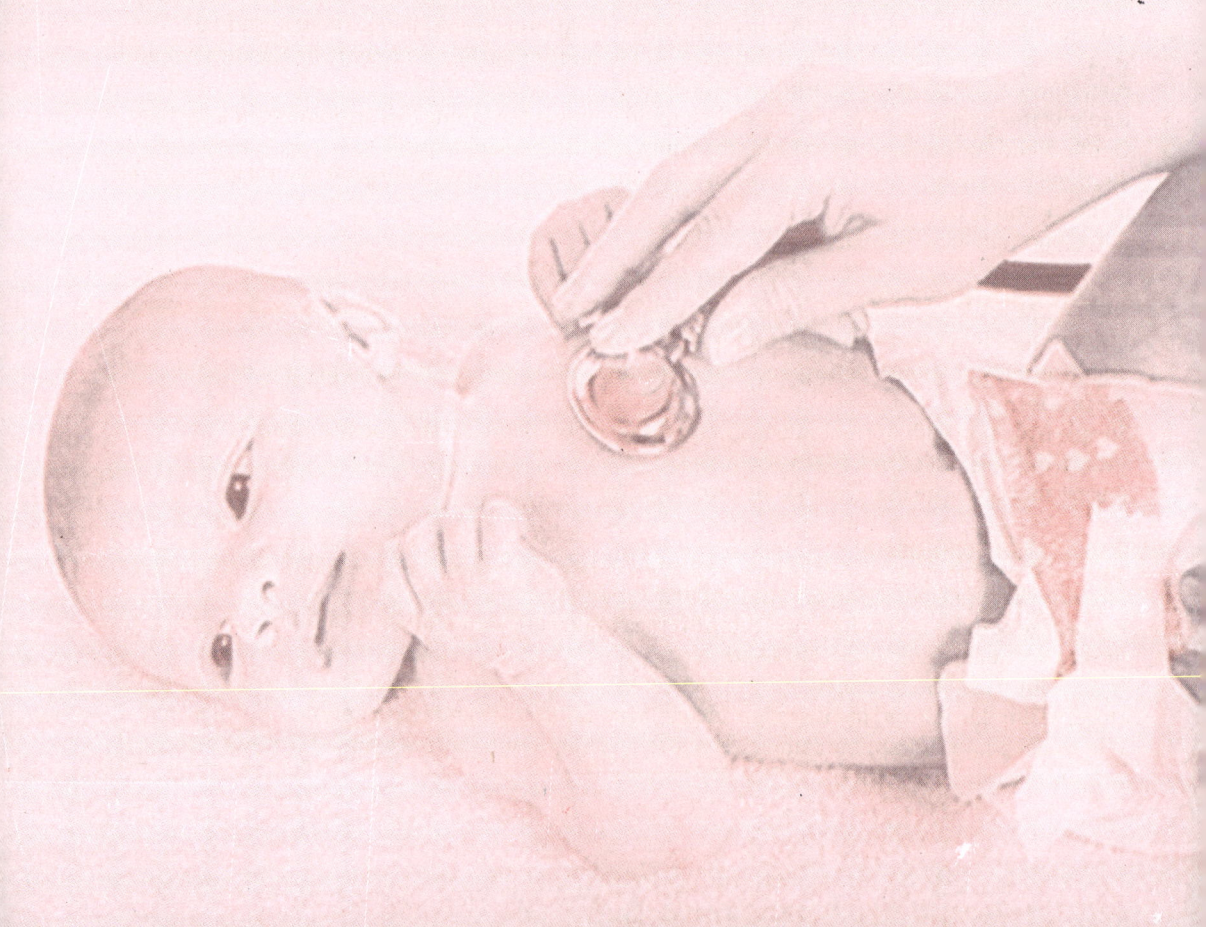

LEARNING OBJECTIVES

On the completion of this chapter, the pediatric nurse will be able to perform the following activities:
- Explain proper preparative care of the child
- Explain the techniques and purpose of suprapubic catheterization

PREOPERATIVE CARE

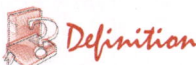 *Definition*

Preoperative care is the preparation and management of a patient prior to surgery. It includes both physical and psychological preparation.

PURPOSES

- For better outcomes
- To reduce fear and anxiety of parents and child
- To alleviate pain
- To prevent postoperative complications

Articles Needed

- Preoperative checklist
- Vitals signs tray
- Surgical clothing
- Consent form
- Child's file
- Weighing scale
- Resuscitation equipment
- Oxygen monitoring system
- Emergency drugs
- Restraints
- Warming devices
- Blanket
- Fluid as prescribed
- Ventilator

PREPARATION OF THE CHILD

Psychological Preparation

- Explain the operation
- Comfort the parents by asking questions
- Give example of other children
- Secure a favorite blanket, toys or other objects to the bed when child is taken to the operating room

- Demonstrate postoperative procedures (deep breathing, coughing and use of blow bottles, turning) have re-demonstration of the procedures
- Assure the parents
- Explain what is NPO sign and stress that child will be fed again as soon as fluid and food can be tolerated
- Discuss means of transportation to operating room and appearance of operating room personnel (colored caps, clothing, mask and gloves)
- Encourage the child to play with mask, caps and gloves.

Physical Preparation

- Medical history and physical examination
- Laboratory investigations
- Monitor vital signs
- Keep the NPO prior to surgery
- Maintain hydration
- Prepare operating site
- Bowel clearance must be there prior to surgery
- Bathe the child and maintain personal hygiene before and on the morning of the surgery
- Urge the child to urinate immediately before medication is given preoperatively
- Administer preoperative medications as per doctor's prescription

PROTECTIVE MEASURES

- Ensure that the consent form is filled up by child's guardian
- All the laboratory reports are included in the chart
- Administer correct dosages of premedications
- Ensure that child's identification band is securely attached
- Have a familiar person stay with the child to provide explanations of strange events and places and to protect him or her physically while awaiting surgery
- Preoperative teaching must be given to prevent postoperative complications
- Give instructions to parents about how to manage the postoperative pain.

PREPARING FOR THE CHILD AND FAMILY FOR SURGERY

Special intervention is needed for a child if child is to undergo a surgical procedure.

Preoperative care for the child who is to undergo surgery is similar to that for adult.

The major difference is that the preparation and teaching must be geared to the child's and developmental level. Presurgical preparation programs allow children and their families to reduce anxiety, knowledge and enhance coping skills.

TABLE 1: Strategies for preoperative teaching

Developmental level	Implications for teaching
Infants and toddlers	• Encourage parents to use a soft tone of voice and stroking and secure, comfortable holding positions to promote calm • Remind parents to use positive facial expressions • Encourage the parents to stay with the child as much as possible

Contd...

Developmental level	Implications for teaching
Preschoolers and school-age children	• Provide explanation • Incorporate pictures and others visual aids in explanation • Ventilate the child about surgery
Adolescents	• Provide detailed explanations • Answers questions honestly

MAINTAINING SAFETY DURING HOSPITALIZATION

Safety is a critical aspect of care of the child in the hospital. Due to their age and developmental level children are vulnerable to harm. Monitor child closely to avoid accidents such as child pushing the knob wrongly, climbing out of the bed, etc. which highlights nursing goals for ensuring safe, developmentally appropriate care for hospitalized child.

POSTOPERATIVE CARE

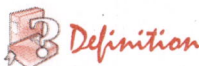 *Definition*

Postoperative care is the management of a patient after surgery. This includes care given during the immediate postoperative period, both in the operating room and postanesthesia care unit

Purposes

- To get better surgical outcomes
- To prevent infection
- To promote healing of surgical incision
- To return the child to normal state of health

PREPARATION

- Prepare the post anesthetic bed prior to shifting from OT
- Assess OT and recovery room records for type of anesthesia, medications and postoperative orders
- Monitor vital signs frequently
- Assess the child's growth and development and level of cognitive functioning
- Determine whether the family members would like to visit the child
- Respect the child's feelings
- Assess the prognosis (activity level, vital signs and skin color)
- Maintain adequate ventilation
- Assess for level of consciousness and feeding
- Pain management
- Do the dressing
- Maintain intake and output chart
- Prevent infection
- Alleviate anxiety
- Prevent complications
- Engage the child with therapeutic play

RESTRAINTS

The restriction often referred to as restraint to ensure safety during therapeutic or diagnostic procedures.

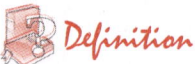 *Definition*

Restraints can be defined as a device to restrict the movements of limbs during therapeutic or diagnostic procedures.

PURPOSE OF RESTRAINTS

- To ensure safety during hospitalization
- To restrict the movements of limbs during diagnostic procedure
- To prevent disruption of prescribed therapy.

TYPES OF RESTRAINTS

- Mummy restraint
- Elbow restraint
- Extremity restraint
- Abdominal restraint
- Jacket restraint
- Mitten or finger restraint

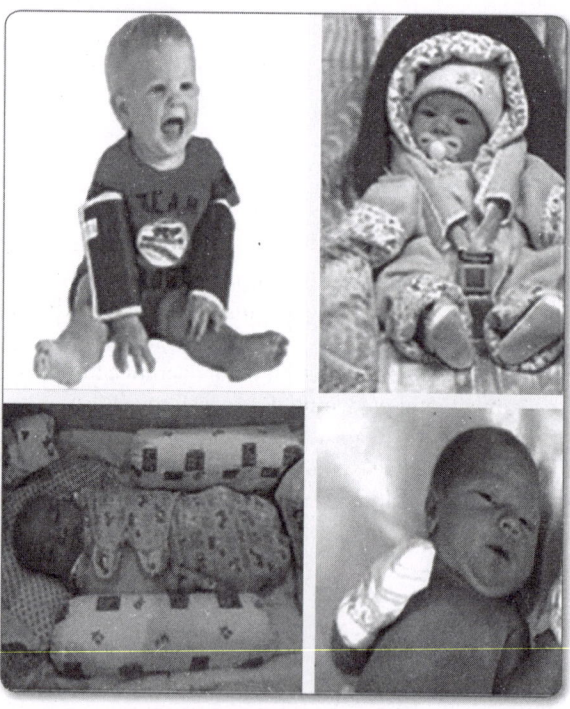

FIG. 1: Types of physical restraints

Mummy Restraint

Body restraint using a sheet folded in a square appropriate to size of the infant or young child to secure the whole body of the child or every extremity except for one.

Safety Concerns

Ensure that all extremities are secured within the sheet.

Elbow Restraint

Prevents child from flexing and reaching face, head, IV and other tubes.

Safety Concerns

Position the restraint so it does not rub against axilla. Check the pulse, temperature and capillary refill of the extremity.

Extremity Restraint

Wrist or ankle restraint to prevent range of motion of extremities.

Safety Concerns

Check wrist or ankle for any sign of circulatory, integumentary or neurologic compromise.

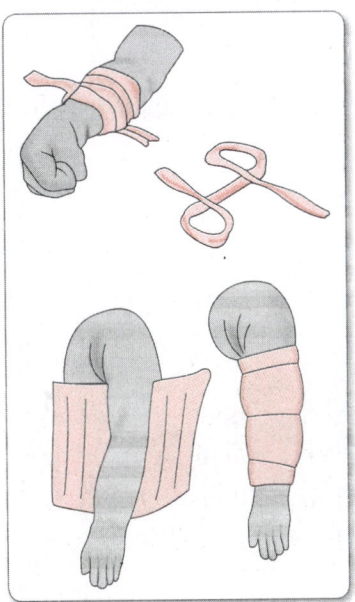

FIG. 2: Wrist or ankle restraint

Jacket Restraint

Jacket worn by child with ties attached to the child's back and to side of bed. Used to keep children flat in bed, such as after surgery or safe in chair.

Safety Concerns

Ensure the child can turn head to side and that the head of the bed is elevated, if possible. Place ties in back so child cannot manipulate them.

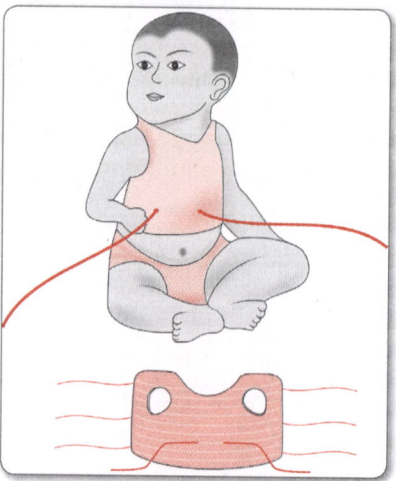

FIG. 3: Jacket restraint

Abdominal Restraint

- This restraint helps to hold the infant in a supine position on the bed.

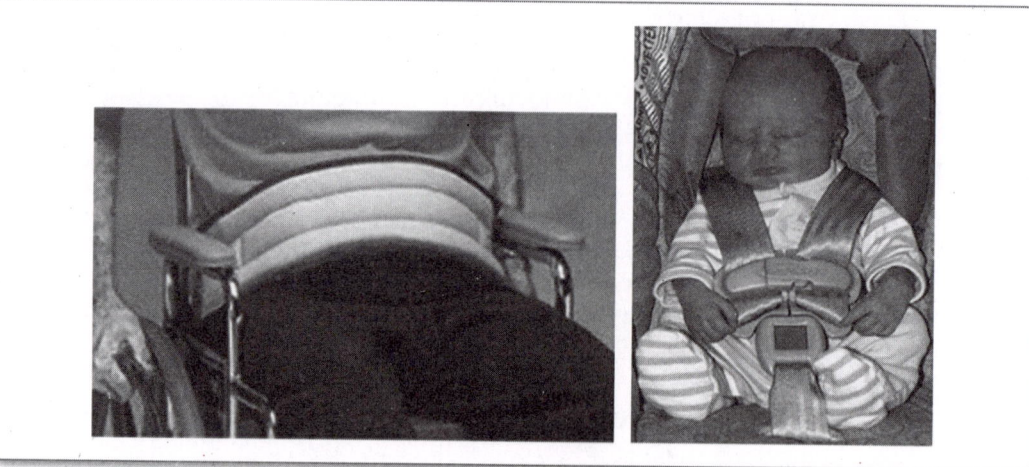

FIG. 4: Abdominal restraint

Mitten or Finger Restraint

- Mitts are used for infants to prevent self-injury by hands in case of burns, facial injury or operations, eczema of the face or body.

- Mitten can be made wrapping the child's hands in gauze or with a little bag putting over the baby's hand and tie it on at the wrist.

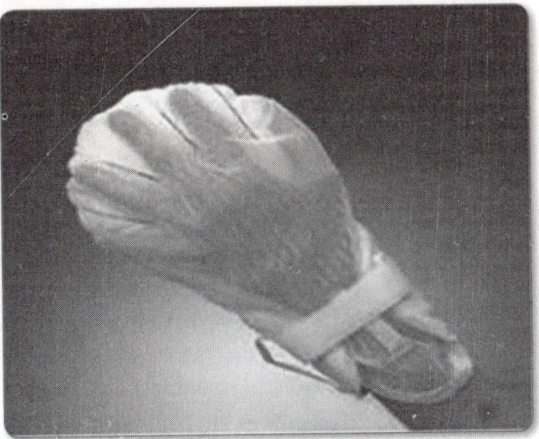

FIG. 5: Mitten restraint

Crib Top Bubble Restraint

Clear plastic cover over the bed to prevent older infant or young child from climbing out of bed and falling.

Safety Concerns

Ensure that there are no tears or loose plastic.

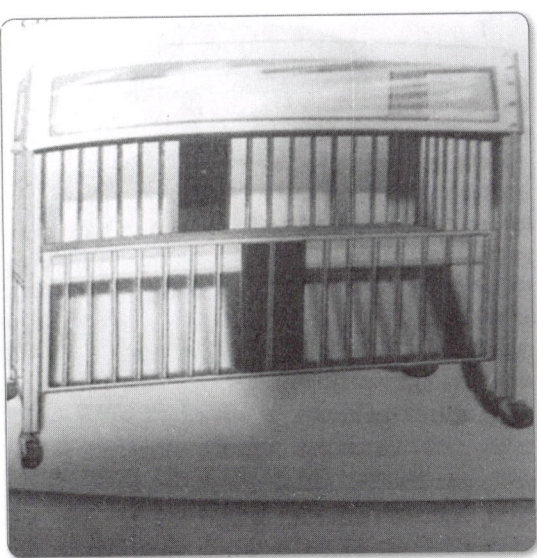

FIG. 6: Crib top bubble restraint

23

Surfactant Therapy

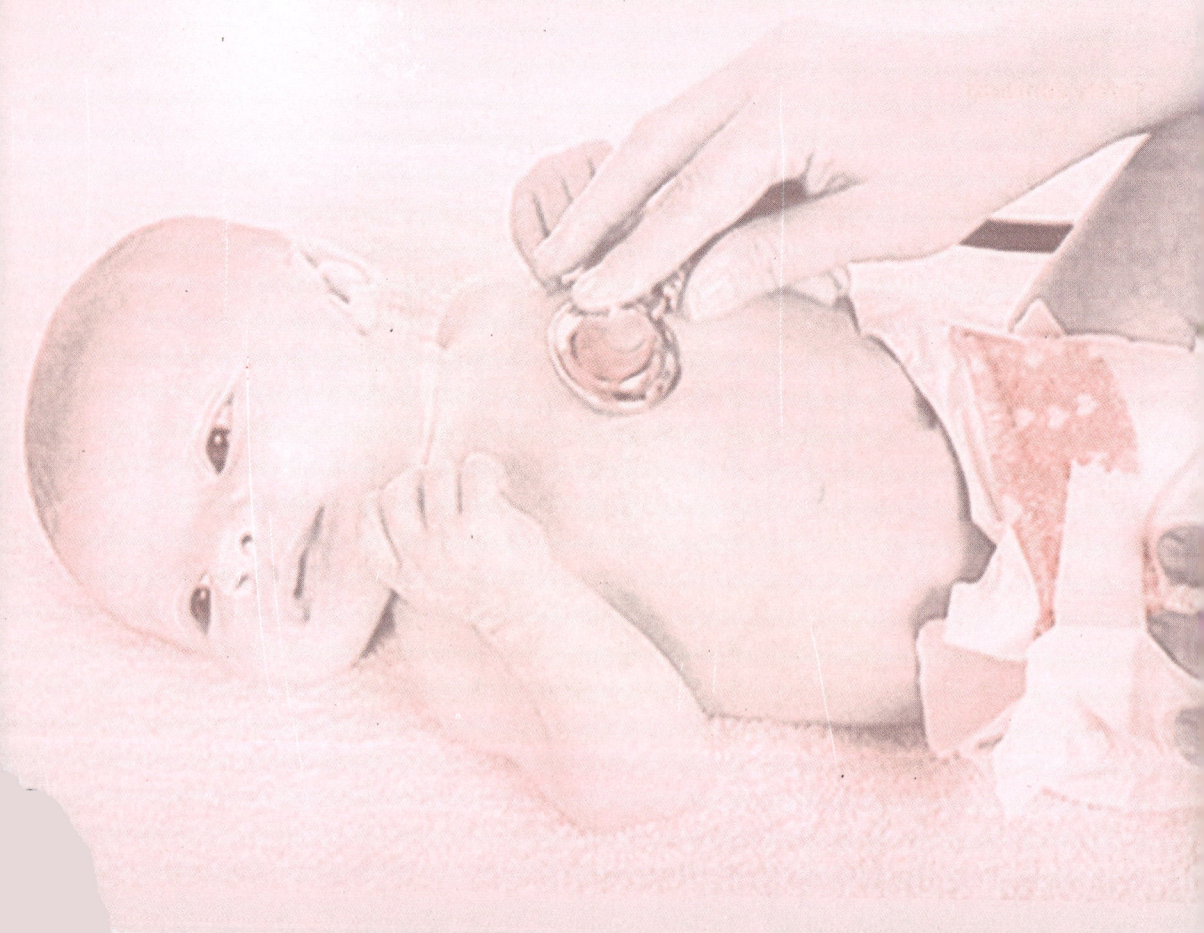

LEARNING OBJECTIVES

On the completion of this chapter, the pediatric nurse would be able to perform the following activity:
- Explain all steps are followed in surfactant therapy

INTRODUCTION

The lungs of preterm infants lack adequate pulmonary surfactant, a constituent of the air liquid surface, that normally with lines the alveolar surfaces and terminal airways. Respiratory distress syndrome (RDS) occurs due to surfactant deficiency, which increases the surface tension at the air–liquid interface of the terminal respiratory units. This leads to atelactasis and increases ventilation perfusion mismatch.

SURFACTANT

Surfactant therapy reduces mortality rates most effectively in infants >30 weeks and those of birth weight >1250 g.

Types

- Synthetic
- Modified natural
- Phospholipids DPPC, animal lung extract
- Spreading agents – acetyl alcohol + tyloxapol, surfactant proteins (SP-B and SP-C)

Procedure

- Surfactant is instilled via tracheal catheterization
- In stable babies with HR > 120 SPO_2 > 85%.
- A 16-gauge vascular catheter is marked to indicate desired depth of insertion (25-26-1 cm) (27-28 weeks 1.5 cm)
- Direct laryngoscopee performed and tracheal catheter was inserted beyond vocal cords and surfactants given at a dose of 100 or 200 mg/kg.

Indications

- Infant at high risk of developing RDS due to short gestation (<32 weeks) or low birth weight <1,300 g)
- Therapeutic administration: Preterm or full-term infants who require endotracheal intubation and mechanical ventilation because of increased work of bathing and increasing O_2 requirements
- Prophylactic therapy: Immediately after birth
- Early rescue therapy: During the 1st few hours after birth
- Continued therapy: Clinical evidence of persistent disease

PERSONNEL

It should be performed under the direction of a physician or by credentilated personnel which include nurses and respiratory therapists

Articles Needed

Administration Equipment

- Syringe containing ordered dose of surfactant, warmed to room temperature
- 5 Fr feeding tube or catheter or endotracheal tube with delivery port
- Mechanical ventilator or resuscitation bag

Resuscitation Equipment

- Laryngoscope and endotracheal tube
- Manual resuscitation bag and airway manometer
- Blended O_2 source
- Suction equipment include catheters, sterile gloves, collecting bottle and tubing and vacuum generator
- Radiant warmer ready for use

Monitoring Equipment

- Neonatal tidal volume monitor, if available
- Airway pressure monitor
- Pulse oximeter or transcutaneous pCO_2
- Cardiorespiratory monitor

Complications

- Plugging of endotracheal tube by surfactant
- Haemoglobin desaturation and increased need for supplemental O_2
- Pharyngeal deposition of surfactant
- Physiologic complications
- Apnea
- Pulmonary hemorrhage from right to left shunting
- Hyperventilation

Procedure

Endotracheal Tube Instillation Using a 5 Fr Catheter

- Insert the pre-cut 5Fr catheter into the endotracheal tube and instill the first half (1.25 mL/kg birth weight) of curosurf
- The infant should be positioned so that either the right or left side is dependent for the dose given
- After the first half is instilled, remove the catheter from the endotracheal tube and manually ventilate the infant with 100 oxygen at a rate of 40–60 breaths/minutes for 1 minute
- When the infant is stable, reposition the infant so that the other side is dependent and administer the remaining half using the same procedures
- Do not suction the infant for at lest 1 hour after administration unless there are signs of significant airway obstruction
- Resume ventilator management and clinical care

24

Chelation Therapy

➲ Chelating Therapy
➲ Blood Gas Analysis

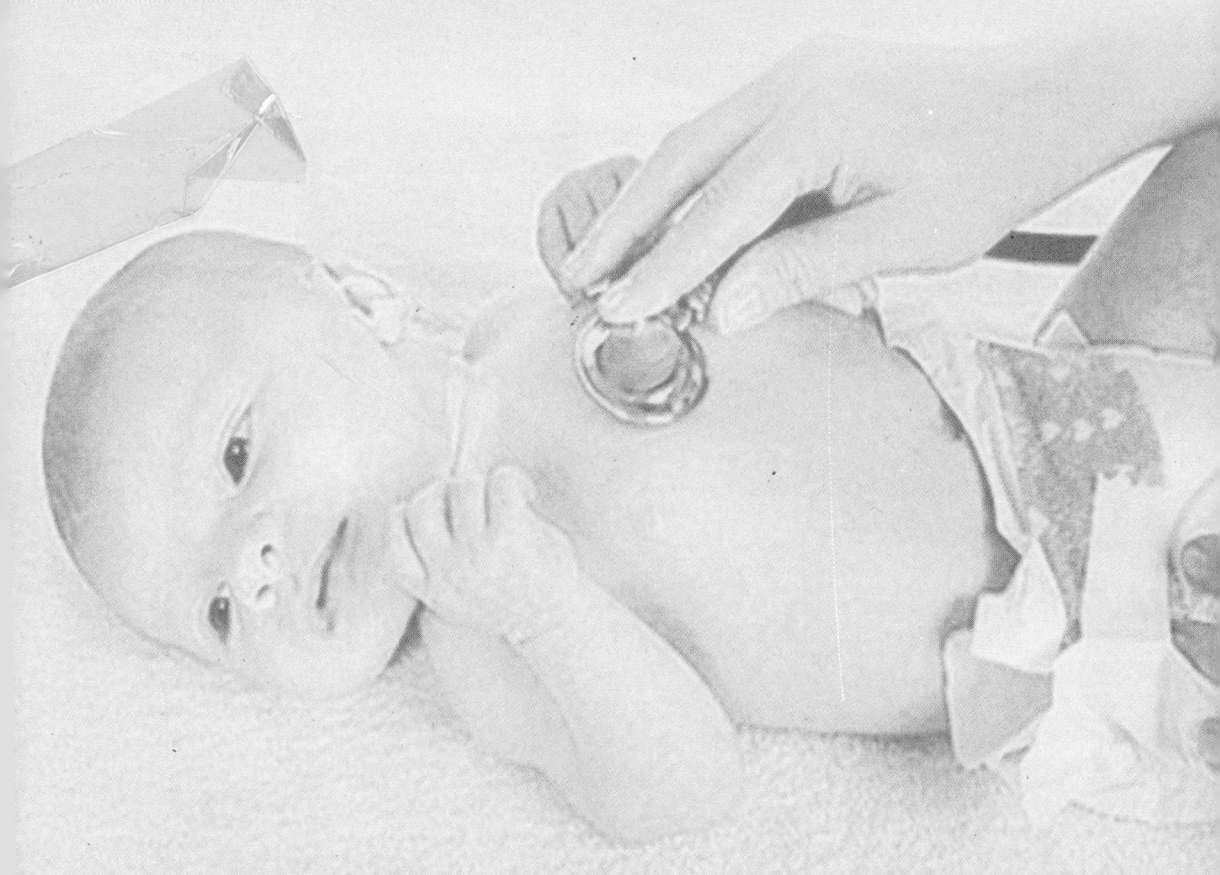

DOSAGE OF CUROSURF

- Intratracheal: Initial: 2.5 mL/kg/dose (200 mg/kg/dose)
- May repeat 1.25 mL/kg/dose (100 mg/kg/dose) at 12-hour intervals for up to 2 additionaly doses, maximum total dose: 5 mL/kg

MANAGEMENT

- Assisted ventilation techniques and O_2 therapy
- Supportive care
  - Thermoregulation
  - Fluid Management
  - Nutrition
  - Antibiotic therapy
- Gentle handling.

LEARNING OBJECTIVES

On the completion of this chapter, the pediatric nurse will be able to perform the following activities:
- Perform chelation therapy
- Perform blood gas analysis

CHELATING THERAPY

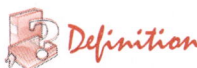 *Definition*

Chelation therapy is the administration of chelating agents to remove heavy metals from the body. It is very helpful in cases of poisoning and the most common form of metal intoxication such as lead, mercury and arsenic poisoning. Chelating agents combine with metals and allow them to be excreted from the body.

Indications of Chelating Therapy
- Mercury poisoning
- Iron poisoning
- Arsenic poisoning
- Lead poisoning
- Uranium
- Plutonium and
- Other forms of heavy metals

Mechanism of Action

The human body is unable to break down heavy metals. When these elements build up and reach toxic levels in the body, it can interfere with the normal functioning of a person. Chelating agents lower the blood levels of metals (e.g. lead, iron, etc.). This is made possible by the attachment of heavy metal molecules to the administered chelating agents. The heavy metal attached to the chelating drugs is then removed from the body through urination. Table enlist common chelating agents

TABLE 1: Common chelating agents

Chelating Agent	Indication for use
Dimercaprol (BAL)	Acute arsenic poisoning Acute mercury poisoning Lead poisoning (with another chelating drug, EDTA)
Edetate calcium disodium or ethylenediamine tetraacetic acid (CaEDTA or EDTA)	Lead poisoning
Deferoxamine	Acute iron poisoning: Iron overload
Dimercaptosuccinic acid (DMSA)	Lead poisoning: Arsenic poisoning and mercury poisoning
Dimercaptopropane sulfonate (DMPS)	Severe acute arsenic poisoning and Severe acute mercury poisoning
Penicillamine	Copper toxicity (mainly used); Adjunct to the therapy in: • Gold poisoning • Arsenic poisoning • Lead poisoning
Succimer (Chemet)	Lead poisoning in pediatric patients with blood lead levels above 45 microgram per decilitre

Side Effects

- Burning sensation at the site of injection or delivery into the vein (common)
- Fever
- Headache
- Nausea
- Stomach upset
- Vomiting
- Flu-like symptoms
- Convulsions
- Bone marrow depression
- Hypotension
- Cardiac arrhythmia
- Respiratory arrest
- Hypocalcemia
- Kidney failure (rare)
- Death (rare)

Contraindications

- Hypersensitivity or known allergy to the drugs

Nursing Implications

- Obtain serum levels of heavy metals (e.g., lead and iron) before the initiation of therapy and again at the termination of the therapy.
- Instruct the parents and child about the need to comply with the full course of medication regimen to achieve desired outcome and effectiveness.
- For EDTA: Monitor serum calcium levels as EDTA removes calcium from the body.
- For EDTA: Injections of EDTA must be given intramuscularly into a large muscle mass. The medication can be combined with 0.5 ml of PROCAINE as the injection of this drug is very painful.
- Measure intake and output to ensure that the kidney is adequately functioning. (If kidney function is not adequate, EDTA may lead to nephrotoxicity or kidney damage).
- Assess the following:
  - BUN
  - Serum creatinine
  - Protein in urine

BLOOD GAS ANALYSIS

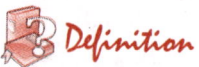 Definition

A blood gas test measures the amount of oxygen and carbon dioxide in the blood. It may also be used to determine the pH of the blood, or how acidic it is. The test is commonly known as a blood gas analysis or arterial blood gas (ABG) test.

Purpose

- To provide a precise measurement of the oxygen and carbon dioxide levels in the body.

- To determine how well the lungs and kidneys are working.
- To identify imbalances in the pH and blood gas levels.
- To monitor treatment for certain conditions, such as lung and kidney diseases.
- To evaluate kidney function.
- To diagnose and evaluate respiratory diseases and conditions.
- To monitor children on oxygen therapy in case of premature infants and children with artificial ventilation.

Indications
- Kidney failure
- Heart failure
- Uncontrolled diabetes
- Hemorrhage
- Chemical poisoning
- A drug overdose
- Shock

Common Sites for Collecting Blood
- Femoral artery
- Dorsalis pedis artery
- **In neonates, capillary blood samples are taken**
- Ulnar and radial artery
- Brachial artery

Articles Needed
- Anticoagulant sterile syringe with needle
- Waste syringe if arterial line draw
- Patient label and laboratory collection slip
- Antiseptic solution
- Gauze pieces
- Pair of sterile gloves
- Personal protective equipment (PPE)
- Container with ice deep enough to immerse syringe beyond the level of specimen

General Instructions
- Psychological preparation should be arranged for child's age and parents.
- The syringe used to collect the sample for a blood gas analysis must contain a small amount of heparin to prevent clotting of the blood.
- Follow the standard precautions for prevention of exposure to blood-borne pathogens when performing arterial blood collection.
- The air must be excluded from the syringe both before and after the sample is collected.
- While transporting the sample, the must be capped with a blind hub, placed on ice and immediately sent to the laboratory for analysis.

- If it is delayed, store the sample in ice (2–4°C).
- Never attempt femoral artery puncture in neonates

Procedure

- Maintain do hand hygiene and put on PPE
- First sterilise the injection site with an antiseptic.
- Insert a needle into the artery and draw blood.
- Seal over the puncture site.
- Expel any air bubbles from the sample and cap the syringe.
- Mix the sample by rolling and tilting syringe.
- The blood sample will then be analyzed by a portable machine or in an on-site laboratory.
- The sample must be analysed within 10 minutes of the procedure to ensure an accurate test result.

Normal Values
- Arterial blood ph: 7.38–7.42
- Bicarbonate: 22–28 milliequivalents per liter
- Partial pressure of oxygen: 75–100 mm hg
- Partial pressure of carbon dioxide: 38–42 mm Hg
- Oxygen saturation: 94–100%

Complications

- Bleeding or bruising at the puncture site
- Feeling faint
- Blood accumulation under the skin
- Infection at the puncture site

25

Play Therapy

LEARNING OBJECTIVES

On the completion of this chapter, the pediatric nurse would be able to perform following activity:
- Provide effective play therapy to the children.

INTRODUCTION

Play is universal for all children. It is work for them and ways of their living. It is pleasurable and enjoyable aspect of a child's life and essential to promote growth and development.

Enjoyment is the essential element in all the play activities. For the child, play is the most essential activity, which serves as a parameter to state whether the child is healthy or underdeveloped or sick or well. It provides valuable learning experience. Play will make the individual or the child to forget his stressful situations and frees them from worries and other stressful responsibilities.

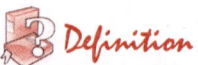 *Definition*

Play is the activity that has no serious motive and from which there is no material gain. The distinction between work and play, however, lies in the mental attitude. Football can be play for children and can be work and means of earning for the professional footballer.

STAGES OF PLAY DEVELOPMENT

Exploratory Stage

From birth to 12 months, infants enjoy or play by seeing at people and objects, make random moments in grasping objects. After gaining voluntary control, a child grasps, holds and examines objects within reach by creeping, crawling and walking.

Toy Stage

The toddler enjoys with toys and feels that their toys have life and capable of acting, talking and feeling. Preschool age children enjoys cooperative and associative play.

Play Stage

- Play becomes a social activity and increases with age, e.g. parallel play, skill play, team games.
- The number of playmates decreases with age, e.g. young children play with anyone whoever is available and willing to play with them. However as age increases, group mates are formed selectively according to their interests.
- As age advances, the child engages in play activities with own sex companions, follows rules and regulations in a formal manner.
- **Play changes from informal to formal:** In childhood the child engages in play activities which are spontaneous and informal, enjoys with toys and with playmates, they do not require any special clothes and equipment.
- A child engages in play activities in a relaxed manner.

- Uses principles of learning to gain experience, e.g. learning by doing, learning by insight, learning by trial and error, learning by conditioning and learning by imitation.
- Play is predictive of the child's personal and social adjustment.
- The child has the opportunity to understand the playmates, behavior.
- School-age children and adolescents enjoy their play by games, sports and hobbies.
- Variations in children play results due to a number of factors such as health, motor development and coordination, intelligence, environment, sex, socioeconomic status, amount of leisure time and playing equipment.

Dream Stage

Adolescents may lose interest in game is and sports depending upon their hobbies, in which they are interested. They enjoy either solitary play or group play.

VALUES OF PLAY

Play is an essential element to development of normal, well adjusted personality in all aspects, i.e. physically, emotionally, mentally, socially and morally through a single type of activity. The child will learn how to adjust in life and play provides a valuable learning experience.

- It is an important tool for socialization; the child tries to learn to understand and communicates with others, enjoys their company and establishes an effective interpersonal relationship through which learns to assume responsibilities.
- The child learns social adjustment patterns; play teaches it children to play adults roles, including sex role behavior.
- Play activities help children to develop muscular coordination, communication skills and senses are exercised; it encourages exploration of physical nature of the ward.
- Helps in maintaining body weight through outdoor games.
- Increases the endurance of the child.
- Fulfils the needs and desires of children by being participants and playing leadership role.
- Acts like a stimulant for creative activities through painting, drawing, clay dolls, puppets, provides an expressive outlet for creative ideas and interests, enhances development of special talents and skills.
- **Self-awareness:** Encourages regulation of own behavior, allows for testing of own abilities; provides for comparison of own abilities with those of others and learns how their own behaviors affects others.
- **Therapeutic values:** Means of outlet for pent-up release of energy to relieve emotional tensions, conflicts and worries; allows for expression of emotions and release of unacceptable impulses in a socially acceptable fashion, encourages experimentation and testing of fearful situation in a safe manner, facilitates nonverbal and communication of needs, fears and desires.
- Develops more definite and realistic concepts of themselves by developing insight into the situations; provides multiple sources of learning, exploration and manipulation of shapes, size, texture and colors, experiences with members, spatial relationships and abstract concepts, it provides opportunity to practice and expand language skills.
- Helps children to understand the world in which they live and to distinguish between reality and fantasy.

- Learns the moral standards, values, procedures and appropriate roles by following the rules, encourages interaction and development of positive attitudes towards others pattern, reinforces approved behavior.
- Makes the child to learn the problem solving approach.
- Desirable personality traits will be acquired, e.g. cooperation, truthful, generous and pleasantness.
- Increases attention, concentration and ability in task-oriented activities and the child learns to control the emotions.
- Child learns the spatial relationships for abstract thinking.
- The child learns to understand the concept of cause and effect and learn to think and solve the problem.
- Develop honesty, sportsmanship and compassion.
- **Speech and language:** Listening to others and family members; saying to others and family members; saying sounds and words, expressing wants and needs while playing. Speaking increases language ability, improves verbal and non-verbal communication, e.g. speech and gestures.
- As the child grows the amount of time spread for play decreases or narrowed and they pursue in other interests and spend their leisure time with those interests.
- Play establishes and maintains emotional balance, enables the child to develop characters such as self control, self-reliance, patience, perseverance, skills and neuromuscular coordination.

TYPES OF PLAY

- **Unoccupied behavior:** Unoccupied behaviour/sense of pleasure play, children from birth to 3 months of age enjoy seeing at others or by random movements, after 3 months to 12 months they the object by holding it. They hand the articles in the environment or by movement of their own bodies by crawling, walking, rocking, with or without support. It represents the lowest extent of social involvement.
- **Social look by at affected play:** An infant tries to maintain their relationships with other people. Adults talk to them, while cuddling and handling them, child responses to adult's talk by smiling or tries to imitate adult's behavior.
- **Solitary independent play:** Plays alone, independent of other children of adults, e.g. one-to-two years of age
- **Outlooker behavior/passive play/amusement:** The child observes others play and will not engage in their play. It is interested in watching various cartoons on TV, listening to stories, poems, radio and music.
- **Parallel play:** It is an independent activity in which the child plays with identical or similar toys which other child plays. Toddlers usually enjoy parallel play.
- **Associative play:** An this activity, all children are engaged in similar type of play activities, whereby social interaction takes place. Child play whatever they want and converse with each other and enjoy the common activity.
- **Cooperative play:** Preschool children play cooperative play and they play with a purpose like preparing a house or making a paper doll. They enjoy the role of leader and participant; share responsibility by assigning tasks to other children.
- **Active play:** Children engage in activities which results in rapid growth of their bodies.
- **Still play:** In this activity action is carried out repeatedly until the child performs well and the skill is attained. Children learns through imitation and in a dramatic manner.

- **Exploratory play:** Young children enjoy exploratory activities, especially male children. When any new toy is given to children, they will try to observe, remove some parts and reassemble and enjoy when it functions again.
- **Constructive play:** Toddlers like to enjoy with building blocks, drawing pictures cartoons
- **Imitative play:** It excites the child's, imagination and improves speaking skill. Children enjoy by learning, identifying themselves with the adults in their environment.
- **Family games:** Infants and toddlers enjoy with their family members during play activities such as hiding an object in one hand and asking the children to identify it, hide seek etc.
- **Neighborhood games:** Preschool children like to enjoy with children from neighbouring houses and spend most of the time there, forming groups playing together.
- **Formal games:** After preschool period and school age, the child loses interests in playing with toys.

CHARACTERISTICS OF PLAY

- Large space is required for different play activities as they need safety, freedom etc. and should provide satisfaction to the child.
- Children enjoy play based on their culture, tradition and background; but it is universal, e.g. young children imitate the play of older children.
- The amount of time children play decreases with age, while other interests increase through years, e.g. toddlers enjoy total time with play alone, preschool age onwards the child has the responsibilities, their interests tend to narrow.
- Play follows a predictable pattern of development.

PLAY MATERIAL TO STIMULATE CHILD DEVELOPMENT

- **For physical development:** Without lessening the pleasure, physical development has to take place simultaneously, e.g. climbing boards, stairs, slides, swing, push and pull toys, see-saw, skates, pools, tricycles, or bicycles, active play.
- **For large muscle coordination:** Engage the child in jumping activities, basket ball, climbing bars, running etc.
- **For small muscle coordination:** Provide crayons, develop drawing skill, painting, peg board, building block
- **For intellectual development:** The child is exposed to his leisure hours in watching educative TV programs, radio, shows, puzzles, games, comics, story books in which children can enrich their intellectual skill.
- **For creative skill:** Providing building blocks, solving puzzle games, clay moulding.
- **Vocabulary development:** Word-building games, comic books and story books expose the child to various educative looks.
  Identify different sounds, objects and freely comment whatever the child feels, encourage him or her to talk in a constructive manner, e.g. allowing the child to participate in debate and quiz programmes.
- **For social development:** Encourage cooperative and associative play. Associate play where the child shares and observes ideas with others and let the child interact with elders and other children, e.g. parents have to teach, guide the child in following norms, manners, customs, traditions and practice good skills along with others.

PLAY IN INFANCY

Motor and sensory development is enhanced with play stimulation. Vocalization is improved as new sounds are learned and sense of trust is developed. Based on the cognitive abilities, play activities should be selected and stimulated at appropriate time. Change in positions by contact with various texture etc, help infants learn to relate to objects and people, to express their feelings and to dispel frustrations through play.

Selection of Play Material in Infancy

- Large toys, where the infant cannot swallow or choke.
- Bright color
- Nontoxic
- Smooth corners
- Rounded edges
- Soft and light weight
- Washable
- If possible, toys should have some sounds, when squeezed.

PLAY IN TODDLER PERIOD

- As attention span is still short, the child tries to concentrate on many activities in a brief period of time
- Gradually, toddlers play activities vary from solitary independent play, on-looker behavior, passive play to parallel play where they may not interact adequately due to inadequate social skill, but they want to be friendly with children.
- When playing with various toys they try to recognize their shapes, colors, sizes, textures, names of the play material.

Types of Game Used

- Rocking horse
- Building block
- Pounding board
- Clay therapy
- Kitchen set
- Mirror
- Crayons
- Hiding behind a tree.

PRESCHOOL PERIOD

- Personality development takes place
- Children develop the ability of children to deal with others
- They are able to express their feelings of anger or love and controls their feelings
- Develop insight and imitation
- Small muscular movement enhances creativity skills among children.

Types of Games Used

- See-saw
- Medium height slide
- Tricycle
- Play cloths for dress up (imitating elders)
- Puzzles

PLAY IN SCHOOL AGE

Play serves as a learning tool and school-age children lives in reality and tries to learn the play activities in a formal, organised and competitive manner. Through fantasy continues and will not share with parent. As the child has interest in learning by doing the things, their attention span increases. Children will develop certain hobbies and acquire knowledge-related facts. They develop the habits of self monitoring and self-evaluation.

Types of Game Used

- Organized games
- Throw games
- Swimming
- Riding cycle
- Musical instruments
- Chess
- Painting
- Snake and ladder
- Video games
- Computer games
- Story books (cartoon, mythical, panchatantra).

PLAY IN PUBESCENT AND ADOLESCENT PERIOD

- Adolescents try out their interests and skills to signify their level of industry
- Learn to work with other and cooperative with each
- Will self-monitor, self-evaluate/judge their own activities
- Will find satisfaction in helping the society
- Makes valuable contributing to social issues
- Level of interests change from games and sports, to computer fields and space sector.

COMMON CAUSES OF IMBALANCE IN PLAY

- **Poor health:** Due to illness, lack of energy occurs and the child may not be able to involve activities. Lack of knowledge of usage of play equipments. Even though the child has variety of play equipment, if the child does not have adequate knowledge related to its usage and operation of its parts, may lead to storage of play equipments alone but not in active use. Parents take initiation and provide an opportunity for the child to learn a variety of play activities and equipment operations.
- **Absence of playmates:** If the playmates are not available, the child's activities are limited to solitary play and it may lead to lack of participation in play, parallel play and social play.

- **Allocation of less time:** The multidimensionality associated with play should be clearly understood by the parents and they encourage the child to involve freely and actively in play activities, as they may be viewed it as a from of activity, a mode or approach to action which results in play behaviour, i.e., it initiates, promotes and sustains learning behaviour. If the parents do not know the values of play and restricts or permits less time, it may affect the all-round personality development of the child.
- **Imbalance between active play and amusements:** Lack of space, increase traffic, over crowding in the urban environment give rise to less chance for the child to involve in active play. Parents encourage children and take them to parks, playground where they can actively participate in different types of play activities. Otherwise, it deprives them of exposure to a wide variety of play activities to discover and meet their play needs. If the parent emphasises on gender-appropriate play activities, it may lead to personal and social maladjustment.
- **Inappropriate selection of play equipment:** The reason such as adult preferences, to little variety of play items, inadequate provision of play equipment according to their age, selecting too simple or too complex or too fragile equipment which may lead to accidents or underutilisation.
- **Absence of practical guidelines to parents or the teachers on play:** Parents and teachers should possess clear-cut guidelines such as how to improvement playway methods. Experts has to conduct training programs and equip both teachers and parents with adequate skills in play activities.

SELECTION OF PLAY MATERIALS

Selection of play materials and toys depends up on age, ability, interests, likes and dislikes, culture, experience, personality and level of intelligence of the child. The play materials should have the following characteristics:

- Safe and washable, light weight, simple, durable, easy to handle and non-breakable
- Realistic, attractive, constructive and offer problem- solving opportunities
- No sharp edges and no small removable parts which may be swallowed or inhaled
- Not overstimulating
- No toxic paints, not costly, not inflammable and not excessive noisy
- Play things with electrical plugs should be avoided, only children over 8 years of age should be permitted to use them
- Toys can be purchased on the basis of safety measures
- Supervision during play is important to prevent accidental injury.

GENERAL INSTRUCTIONS FOR PLAY THERAPY

- The nurse must consider the age, interest, diagnosis, conditions and limitations of the child imposed by doctors when planning activities for any child
- When using play as a part of nursing care, it is important to evaluate the outcome of play
- Explain the importance of play to parents and children
- Special consideration must be given to the child who is isolated, has limited movements or restricted extremities.
- Nurse must perform special activities during special procedures in case of oral fluid intake, injections, deep breathing and range of motion and use of extremities
- Award the child when he or she completes activities
- Teach the child to take care of their toys
- Sessions can include a range of activities, which are usually chosen based on the child's age and preference.

26

Care of a Child with Plaster Cast

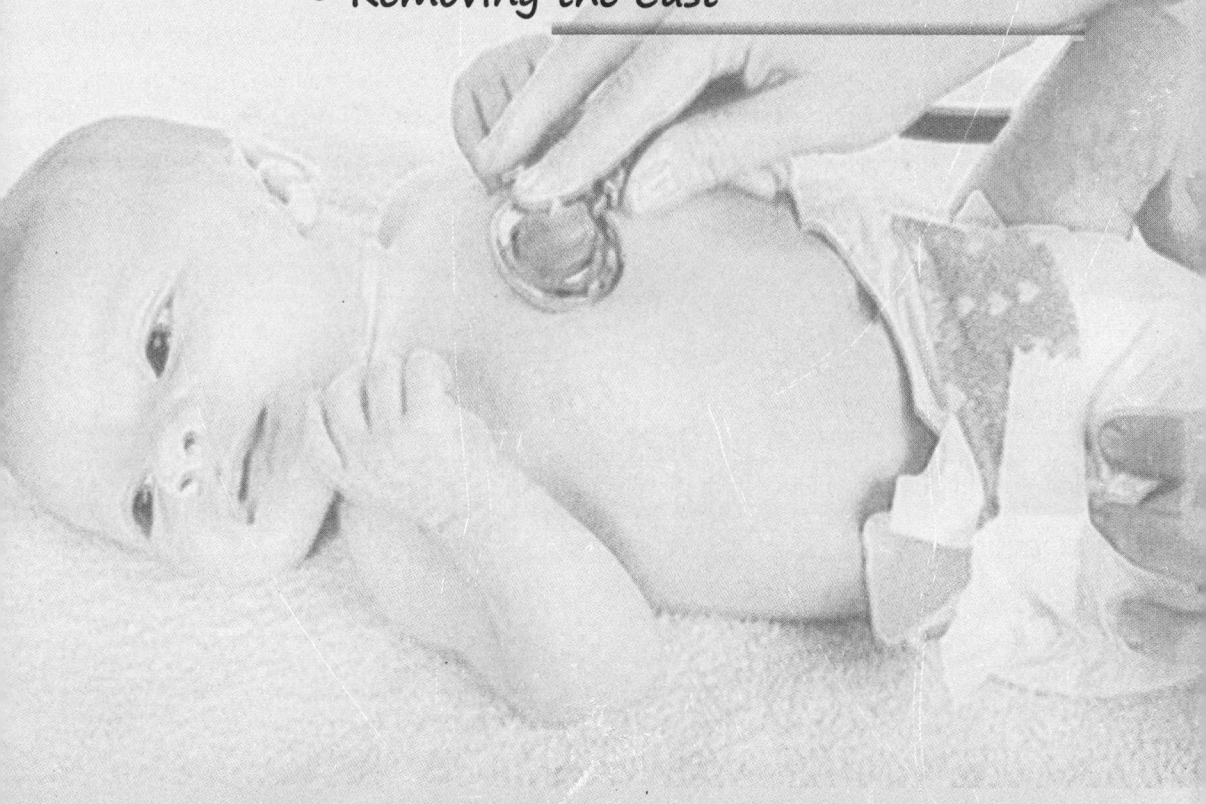

LEARNING OBJECTIVES

On the completion of this chapter, the pediatric nurse would be able to perform the given activity:
- Provide care to the child with plaster cast

INTRODUCTION

A plaster cast is applied to hold the arm or leg fracture in place while the bone heals. On average, plaster casts stay on for about 6 weeks.

PURPOSES

- To prevent the bones from moving
- To realign bone fragments
- To provide rest and heal
- To correct deformity
- To treat dislocation
- To reduce muscle spasms

Points to Remember

- Rest the plaster on something soft until it dries; use a pillow to rest the child's limb on
- Do keep the plaster raised especially for 24–48 hours, to prevent swelling; elevate the leg on pillows initially and at night
- Ensure the child frequently exercises his or her toes
- Do check the color of the child's toes – they should be pink; squeeze the nail white, then release. They should return immediately to pink
- Do watch for swelling – when the child hangs his or her leg down, there will be some swelling. Get them to rest their leg on a chair for a couple of hours – compare it to the other leg; are they the same?
- Do keep your cast clean and dry
- Do check around the plaster for any smells – plasters do have a slight smell but should not be unpleasant
- Don't press on the plaster for 24–48 hours until dry; pressing on it will dent it
- Don't poke anything, such as knitting needles, down the plaster; it may damage your child's skin
- Don't let the child walk on their plaster:
  - Without using crutches
  - Without instructions from the doctor
- Don't put lotions, creams or powder inside the plaster or around the edges

Articles Needed Used

- Gauze strips and bandages impregnated with plaster of paris
- Synthetic light weight, water-resistant materials (e.g., fiberglass and polyurethane resin)

TYPES OF CASTS

- Long leg cast
- Short leg cast

- Bilateral long leg cast
- Full spica cast
- Single spica
- Short-arm cast
- Long-arm cast

PREPARATION BEFORE THE PROCEDURE

Assess baseline neurovascular assessment:
- Color (note cyanosis or other discoloration)
- Movement (note inability to move finger or cast)
- Sensation (note of sensation is present)
  - Edema

QUALITY OF PULSES

- Premedication as ordered to reduce pain.
- Child will be brought into the X-ray room and asked to stay still while a special camera takes a picture of the bones in the injured minutes.

DURING THE PROCEDURE

- A cast is essentially a big, hard bandage that keeps a bone from moving during the healing process. It generally has two layers: A soft layer of padding that rests against the skin and a hard outer layer that protects the bone.
- Doctors sometimes make tiny cuts in the sides of a cast so that there is room for swelling if it occurs.

STEPS OF PROCEDURE

Step/task
Identify the child
Greet the child and the family members
Introduce self and the procedure to be performed
Check for the circulatory, neurological integrity around the cast already applied. • Paleness • Cyanosis • Unusual coldness • Mottled appearance • Tingling or numbness • Pain or burning sensation • Weak or absent peripheral pulse • Ability to move toes of fingers
Check for any sign of infection or swelling around the cast
Assess for the tightness of the cast by inserting finger between the skin and the cast (after it is dried well)
Assess the child's respiratory rate and depth, color and behavior are assessed

Contd...

Step/task
Assess the vitals of the patient
Trim the rough edges of the plaster
Provide required padding
Inspect the cast again for any small objects beneath the cast and any hot spot
Check for the dryness of the cast. If not dry allow adequate position change to dry it
Check for the color and cleanliness of the cast; if not clean or soiled, apply white shoe polish to clean it and dry
Provide active and passive exercises; if the child is in body spica, or in hip spics, he/she should be turned routinely
Support the uncasted areas of the body with pillows
Instruct the child and the parents not to try inserting any object on using lotion or powder on the skin beneath the cast
Teach the parents how to care for the child in a cast and sign and symptoms of the circulatory and neurosensory impairment and infection.

AFTER THE PROCEDURE

- The first few days, when the children in the cast are often the most difficult time for both parents and the child.
- The area surrounding the fracture is probably still sore and swollen.
- The doctor may recommend acetaminophen or ibuprofen to help alleviate any pain.
- The doctor may also recommend
  - Elevating the limb: Use something soft, like a pillow to raise the injured arm or leg above the heart to reduce swelling.
  - Icing: Put ice in a plastic bag, and then place the bag over the injured area.
- If the cast or splint is on an arm, the nurse or technician will give the child a sling to help support it. A sling is made of cloth and a strap that loops around the back of the neck and acts like a special sleeve to keep the arm comfortable and in place. A child with a broken leg who is mature enough will probably get crutches to make it a little easier to get around.
- Sometimes a 'walking cast' (a foot or leg cast with a special device implanted in the heel to allow for walking) can be given, though your child shouldn't walk on it until it is dry.

CAST-CARE TIPS

These tips can help ensure your child's cast stays in good shape:
- Keep non-waterproof casts dry
- Keep out foreign objects or substances.
- Check for cracks.
- Don't alter the cast.

WHEN TO CALL THE DOCTOR?

- Increased pain that is not better with ice, elevation, and/or pain medication
- Extreme tightness that leads to the hand or foot feeling numb or tingly
- Fingers or toes turning white, purple or blue

- Loss of movement of toes or fingers
- A blister developing inside the cast
- Any unusual odour or drainage coming from inside the cast
- A break in the cast or the cast becoming loose
- Skin around the edges of the cast getting red or raw
- Fever

REMOVING THE CAST

Once the bone is healed, the cast will be removed with a small electrical saw. The saw's blade is not sharp—it has a dull, rounded edge that vibrates from side to side. This vibration is strong enough to break apart the fiberglass or plaster but should not hurt the child's skin. Once the cast is off, the injured area will probably look and feel different to the child. The skin will be pale, dry, or flaky; the hair will look darker; and the muscles in the area will look smaller or thinner. This is all temporary.

NOTES